Updates in Clinical Dermatology

Updates in Clinical Dermatology aims to promote the rapid and efficient transfer of medical research into clinical practice. It is published in four volumes per year. Covering new developments and innovations in all fields of clinical dermatology, it provides the clinician with a review and summary of recent research and its implications for clinical practice. Each volume is focused on a clinically relevant topic and explains how research results impact diagnostics, treatment options and procedures as well as patient management. The reader-friendly volumes are highly structured with core messages, summaries, tables, diagrams and illustrations and are written by internationally well-known experts in the field. A volume editor supervises the authors in his/her field of expertise in order to ensure that each volume provides cutting-edge information most relevant and useful for clinical dermatologists. Contributions to the series are peer reviewed by an editorial board.

Esraa M. AlEdani • Howard I. Maibach
Editors

Applications of Artificial Intelligence in Common Dermatological Diseases

Springer

Editors
Esraa M. AlEdani
University of Basrah, College of Medicine
Basra, Iraq

Howard I. Maibach
University of California - San Francisco
San Francisco, CA, USA

ISSN 2523-8884 ISSN 2523-8892 (electronic)
Updates in Clinical Dermatology
ISBN 978-3-031-78138-4 ISBN 978-3-031-78139-1 (eBook)
https://doi.org/10.1007/978-3-031-78139-1

This Springer imprint is published by the registered company Springer Nature Switzerland AG
The registered company address is: Gewerbestrasse 11, 6330 Cham, Switzerland

To the patients

Whose experiences, conditions, and stories lie at the heart of every image, every dataset, and every line of code.

Your silent resilience and willingness to contribute to the advancement of medical knowledge are the foundation of this work.

To the pioneers of artificial intelligence

Whose bold imaginations have shaped technologies that were once the stuff of science fiction and are now transforming lives.

To the dermatologists and clinicians

Who recognize the value of innovation and embrace change not as a threat, but as a tool to enhance care, equity, and accuracy.

And most personally, to my family

Thank you for being my source of balance, strength, and endless encouragement. Your love made this journey possible.

And finally to myself who spent an uncountable amount of hours putting all my blood, sweat, and tears into this book.

Preface

The advent of artificial intelligence (AI) has ushered in a new era of innovation and transformation across numerous disciplines, with dermatology standing at the forefront of these advancements. This compilation of chapters delves into the multifaceted role that AI plays in modern dermatology, from the early detection of skin cancers and prediction of skin sensitization to the management of chronic conditions like psoriasis. The integration of AI into dermatological practice promises to enhance diagnostic accuracy, improve patient outcomes, and potentially revolutionize the way skin diseases are treated and managed.

This work begins by providing a historical context, tracing the evolution of AI from its theoretical origins to its current applications in dermatology. The chapters explore the technical underpinnings of AI, including convolutional neural networks (CNNs) and machine learning models, and their specific applications in diagnosing skin conditions. A significant portion of the text is dedicated to examining AI's role in skin cancer detection, where it has shown remarkable accuracy in identifying malignant lesions, sometimes surpassing the capabilities of seasoned dermatologists.

However, the promise of AI is not without its challenges. This collection also addresses the various obstacles that hinder the seamless integration of AI into clinical practice. These include issues of data standardization, the representativeness of training datasets, and the ethical implications of AI-driven diagnostics. The underrepresentation of diverse skin tones in AI research poses a significant risk of exacerbating existing healthcare disparities. The text also critically examines the limitations of AI in clinical settings, highlighting the importance of combining AI with traditional diagnostic methods to ensure comprehensive patient care.

In addition to the clinical applications, this work explores AI's role in predicting skin sensitization, an area of growing importance given the ethical and regulatory pressures to move away from animal testing. The discussion covers the use of in silico models, deep learning techniques, and integrated approaches that combine multiple methods to enhance predictive accuracy.

As AI technology continues to evolve, it holds the potential to not only transform dermatology but also redefine the broader healthcare landscape. The text envisions a future where AI-driven tools are integral to clinical decision-making, leading to more personalized and effective treatments. Yet, it also underscores the necessity for ongoing research, ethical considerations, and the development of robust regulatory frameworks to guide the responsible use of AI in medicine.

This compilation is intended for a broad audience, including dermatologists, medical researchers, data scientists, and students. It aims to provide a comprehensive understanding of the current state of AI in dermatology, the challenges that lie ahead, and the opportunities for future advancements. By offering a balanced perspective on the promise and pitfalls of AI, this work seeks to contribute to the ongoing dialogue about how best to harness this powerful technology for the benefit of patients and the field of dermatology as a whole.

Basra, Iraq — Esraa M. AlEdani
San Francisco, CA, USA — Howard I. Maibach

Acknowledgments

This book is the product of years of study, collaboration, and research across multiple disciplines. I am deeply grateful to the institutions that nurtured this project from its earliest stages to its final form. Special thanks to [Springer—Updates in Clinical Dermatology], whose support for interdisciplinary innovation allowed for a meaningful convergence of technology and medicine and who eased the process.

No work of scholarship is ever completed in isolation, and I owe an enormous debt of gratitude to my mentors and advisors. Foremost, I would like to thank Dr. Howard Maibach, whose mentorship has been a guiding light. Your insights challenged me to think critically, work methodically, and write responsibly. You saw potential where I saw uncertainty, and for that, I am profoundly grateful.

To all the professors and guest lecturers who contributed knowledge, editing it and guidance, and feedback throughout the years—thank you for pushing me to go beyond surface-level inquiry and embrace the complexity that comes with meaningful research.

This work represents a collaborative effort across numerous domains and professionals. To the clinical researchers, dermatology residents, and attending physicians who provided annotations, feedback, and case validation—you brought clinical realism and relevance to this research. Your knowledge grounded the theoretical aspects of AI in real-world scenarios.

To the data scientists, machine learning engineers, and research assistants who worked with me to build, test, and refine models—thank you for your patience, your commitment to quality, and your creativity. Long hours of training data, countless code iterations, and versioning trials were all worth it because of your dedication.

Special thanks also go to the contributors from open-source platforms and medical AI communities who have been generous with data, code, and peer support. This project is part of a larger collective movement, and I am grateful to be part of it.

I want to take this space to recognize the patients whose anonymized data formed the foundation of many experiments and validations presented in this book. Your trust in research, your openness in sharing clinical records, and your courage to contribute—often without knowing who would benefit or when—have helped shape the future of dermatological care.

This book is written in honor of your experiences and in pursuit of reducing misdiagnosis, improving access, and accelerating clinical responses. I hope the ideas shared here will eventually translate into better, faster, and more personalized dermatologic treatments for others like you.

Equally, I extend appreciation to the ethics boards and privacy officers who helped ensure that this work was carried out with the highest regard for patient confidentiality, data responsibility, and human dignity.

To my family—words will never fully capture the gratitude I feel. Your patience through late nights, your encouragement during self-doubt, and your belief in my work were the quiet forces that kept me going. To my parents, thank you for your sacrifices and for instilling in me a curiosity that knows no bounds. To my mother, Feryal Abbas, your presence was a refuge. Your steady confidence in my abilities reminded me daily of what really matters and of what I deserve in my life.

To my friends and peers—thank you for the laughter, for distracting me when I needed a break, and for challenging me to return to the work with fresh eyes.

Finally, to the future:

As this book considers the first one which combines AI and Dermatology. May this book be a small but meaningful contribution to a growing field. May it inspire new questions, spark thoughtful debate, and serve as a resource to those who strive to integrate artificial intelligence responsibly into dermatology. The journey is far from over, but if this work serves as a useful step forward, then it has fulfilled its purpose.

Contents

The Role of AI in Dermatology

1

Esraa M. AlEdani

1.1 Overview

Artificial intelligence (AI) is a computer science that aims to replicate human intellect and analyze complicated data. This notion is widely thought to have originated during the 1956 Dartmouth Conference. However, the technology available at the time limited the use of AI.

Significant gains in processing power have occurred recently as a result of better hardware and software technologies. AI is becoming recognized for its potential to enhance procedures in several areas, including medicine. Dermatology is in a unique position to be an early candidate for AI deployment due to its extensive clinical imaging databases for use and interpretation. Dermatologists will need to grasp the fundamentals of AI in order to develop and analyze medical investigations in this field. As a result, this analysis begins with an overview of AI procedures. It will then continue on to explore the current literature on the use of AI in dermatology. Finally, it will address any potential problems with this technology.

1.2 Brief History of AI

Computer scientists produced code to decode the German Enigma code during World War II, which is when artificial intelligence (AI) was first used. Despite the lack of a title for it, these developments set the foundation for machine learning (ML) and artificial intelligence. The creation of expert systems that could execute mathematical algorithms quickly was a major advance between 1950 and 1980. Notably, in 1951, the Ferranti Mark 1 computer used algorithms to become a

E. M. AlEdani (✉)
University of Basrah, College of Medicine, Basra, Iraq

E. M. AlEdani, H. I. Maibach (eds.), *Applications of Artificial Intelligence in Common Dermatological Diseases*, Updates in Clinical Dermatology,
https://doi.org/10.1007/978-3-031-78139-1_1

master of checkers. It wasn't until 1956—during a Dartmouth computer science conference—that computer and cognitive scientist John McCarthy (1927–2011), who was practicing artificial intelligence, officially named the field. Following the term's debut, mathematical and geometric algorithms were developed in the 1960s, which resulted in the creation of WABOT-1, the first humanoid robot and the beginning of physical artificial intelligence. Even with sufficient funding, the capabilities of computers at the time severely limited AI efforts. A new wave of excitement was brought about between 1985 and 2005 as a result of advancements in neural networks, logistic regression, K-nearest neighbors, probabilistic modeling, and decision trees.

The Japanese government revealed aspirations to create a computer that could perform sophisticated machine learning in the late 1990s.

IBM created Deep Blue, the first artificial intelligence algorithm to beat a global chess champion, not long after. Despite the progress, the early 2000s' dotcom boom crashed and a lack of finance caused a further standstill. Ten major corporations are now developing technologies using new AI techniques. Examples of these include Tesla's self-driving cars (Palo Alto, CA) and Amazon's Alexa (Seattle, WA) and Google Translate (Mountain View, CA).

When dermatopathologic diagnoses were produced in 1987 using microcomputer systems, it was one of the first times artificial intelligence (AI) was mentioned in the field of dermatology. Not too long after, dermatologists could now get help from computers for prognostication, diagnosis, and literature searches. Melanomas, nonmelanoma skin cancer, vitiligo, and atopic dermatitis were among the conditions for which artificial neural networks (ANNs) (described later in this paper) and pattern recognition were investigated in the 2000s. AI-based diagnostic systems have been developed by numerous teams and studies in recent years, and some of them have shown to be on par with or even superior to small cohorts of board-certified dermatologists. As of right now, the US Food and Drug Administration has not authorized any AI systems related to dermatology.

1.3 AI Popularity

Despite being present for more than 50 years, artificial intelligence has just lately become widely recognized. Artificial intelligence (AI) systems are highlighted in movies and television series including The Terminator, iRobot, Westworld, and Black Mirror. These media also encourage dialogue about real-world and imaginary AI uses, as well as the ethical and social issues surrounding AI technology. Furthermore, businesses like Waltham, Massachusetts-based Boston Dynamics have brought previously imaginary humanoids to life with their quadruped and biped robots, which have been seen in films carrying out a range of human activities. Even well-known people have weighed in on the development of AI, with Elon Musk, Stephen Hawking, and Bill Gates among them cautioning about the risks associated with super AI systems.

1.4 AI in Medicine

The idea that AI could eventually take the role of doctors has drawn more interest to AI in medicine; however this is extremely unlikely. The most likely result is that AI will be used as a supplement to assist medical professionals in sorting through information and making more informed decisions. AI's capacity to "learn" from enormous databases of dermatological and medical information is proof of this. It's noteworthy to note that, despite uncertainty about how, modern systems are acknowledged to be self-correcting. The future applications of artificial intelligence (AI) and machine learning are not fully known, but this uncertainty is probably contributing to the technology's continued appeal.

1.5 Basic Knowledge of Artificial Intelligence (AI)

Although AI may be classified in a variety of ways, it is often divided into two subcategories: strong AI and weak AI. A machine with human-level intelligence is referred to as "strong AI" or "artificial general intelligence." This often refers to a complicated machine that has learned to do a variety of activities on its own and has the ability to learn new ones. This wide category includes computers capable of awareness, ethical cognition, and multitasking. Currently, powerful artificial intelligence is mostly seen in science fiction and popular culture. In contrast, weak or narrow AI refers to existing technology in which a computer learns to achieve a purpose. To execute different jobs with weak AI, various programs are required.

1.5.1 Machine Learning

Machine learning (ML) is an approach for developing artificial intelligence. Machine learning involves computer programs generating their own code to complete a predefined goal. This method can be either monitored, semi-supervised, or unsupervised. Supervised learning involves labeling each sample in a dataset with a specific response. The system then learns by trial and error to predict the answer from the input dataset. Unsupervised learning is the processing of input data with no defined answer. This technique is frequently used to simulate data structures and distribution. Semi-supervised learning combines both labeled and unlabeled data. This can assist in alleviating the load of labeling as shown in Fig. 1.1.

1.5.2 Deep Learning

Whereas ML is the capacity of machines to automate a learning process, deep learning (DL) refers to a specific sort of ML that employs artificial neural networks (ANNs). This type of machine learning allows for an infinite number of layers, with

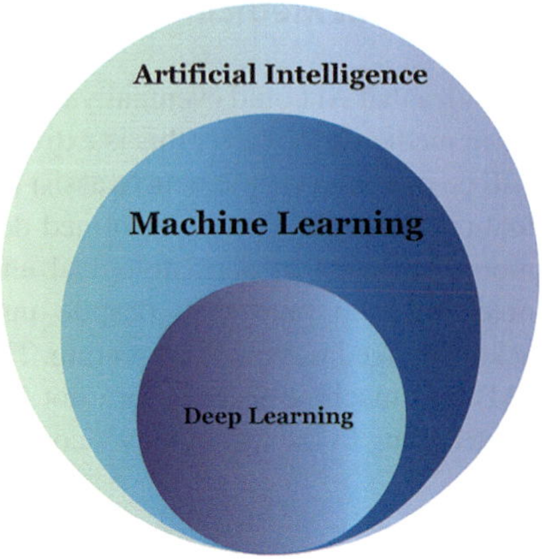

Fig. 1.1 An overview of the correlation of AI, ML, and DL

each layer able to identify and learn unique dataset-specific properties. The model's multiple-layered structure enables it to learn complicated tasks.

1.5.3 Evaluating Artificial Intelligence Programs

Dermatologists are familiar with many statistical measures, such as sensitivity and specificity, that are frequently used to evaluate AI programs. However, the area under the receiver operating characteristic curve (AUROC) is a statistical metric that is frequently used to assess AI programs and may not be familiar to all dermatologists. The ability of a test to distinguish between two states—typically, "disease" and "no disease"—is measured by the AUROC. An AUROC of 1.00 and perfect discrimination are implied by the complete separation of accurate classification from misclassification. If the outcome is 0.5, it means that the findings are just grouped based on chance.

1.6 Applications of AI in Dermatology

Numerous uses of AI exist in dermatology and medicine. AI is currently being used in medicine for a variety of purposes, such as illness diagnosis and treatment, population health interventions, physician tools, insurance, patient-based diagnostics and education, and data infrastructure powering. Although AI systems can now distinguish between information that is useful and irrelevant on their own, they still need to be trained on a collection of data before they can learn on their own. These consist of genetics, electrodiagnosis, physiologic monitoring, diagnostic imaging, evaluation of disability, and mass screening. The applications are extensive and have the ability to consistently deliver current information, lower treatment and diagnostic errors, and tailored patient outcomes based on unique risk factors. While many of

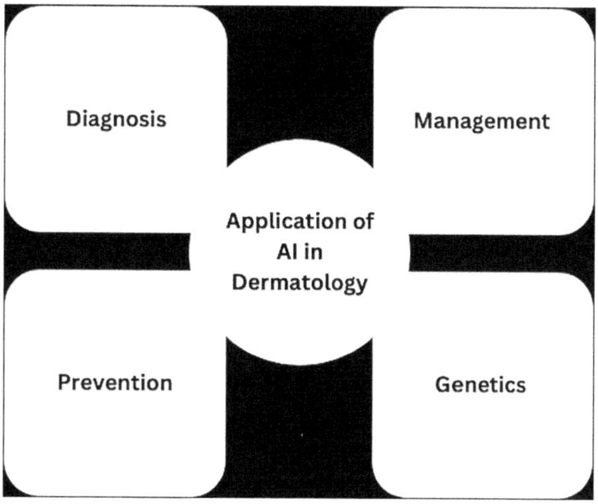

Fig. 1.2 General application of AI

the technologies presented are not widely used by dermatologists, the following applications might be used in the future, as shown in Fig. 1.2.

1.6.1 Diagnostics

Change is one of the most crucial traits used to identify a melanoma. Patients can snap photos of skin lesions and monitor them over time with the use of mole tracker applications like MoleMapper. Dermatologists can view these photos and compare them to earlier ones to find any changes in size or color that might point to a melanoma diagnosis. Patients can also use other mobile applications to transmit photographs to a dermatologist, make appointments for dermatology, and get a differential diagnosis and treatment plan for their lesion. This gives customers a great deal of independence when it comes to their dermatological care. There are issues with the veracity of these apps, even when they provide disclaimers. Users should consult a dermatologist and use skepticism toward the results, should they be worried about a lesion.

1.6.2 Management

Information is spreading at a never-before-seen pace. As more and more material is produced, we may be producing a data overload where new discoveries are not immediately incorporated into dermatology practice, leading to the eventual emergence of a knowledge gap. Additionally, because of this information gap, new therapies are adopted more slowly, which eventually costs the patient. NLP may need to be used in order to help with patient management due to this discrepancy. For instance, the "Oncology Expert Advisor" is meant to act as a management advisor, offer treatment recommendations, and summarize a patient's medical history. By compiling and summarizing patient data, this system is an effective tool that has the potential to reduce wait times and enhance patient care. Such technologies are capable of assessing each patient individually and providing relevant recommendations. In addition to management, AI systems can provide personalized prognostic assessments and result forecasts. Examples from cardiology and oncology are numerous.

1.6.3 Preventive Medicine

AI systems are not yet commonly used in dermatological practice and have received little validation. Algorithms could play a big part in preventive medicine as they continue to advance. Artificial intelligence (AI) algorithms may be able to provide tailored recommendations based on individual risk variables.

Primary, secondary, and tertiary prevention are the three categories of preventive medicine; the last is the least cost-effective. Primary and secondary prevention offer substantial cost savings. Clinical preventative services cost patients considerable time and are underutilized. In other disciplines, like cardiology, AI-based primary and secondary preventive strategies are now being researched. Dermatologists will have a reliable way to offer prompt and precise preventive advice once AI models are put into practice.

1.6.4 Genetics

Numerous works on AI and genomics have been published. These studies include a wide range of topics, such as the identification of genes, splice sites, exons, transcription start sites, and gene function prediction. There is a chance to identify genes that could be implicated in the development of skin cancer and other dermatologic diseases through the limited number of AI studies about dermatologic genomics.

References

1. Hogarty DT, Su JC, Phan K, et al. Artificial intelligence in dermatology—where we are and the way to the future: a review. Am J Clin Dermatol. 2020;21:41–7. https://doi.org/10.1007/s40257-019-00462-6.
2. Du-Harpur X, Watt FM, Luscombe NM, Lynch MD. What is AI? Applications of artificial intelligence to dermatology. Br J Dermatol. 2020;183(3):423–30. https://doi.org/10.1111/bjd.18880. Epub 2020 Mar 29. PMID: 31960407; PMCID: PMC7497072
3. Young AT, Xiong M, Pfau J, Keiser MJ, Wei ML. Artificial intelligence in dermatology: a primer. J Invest Dermatol. 2020;140(8):1504–12. https://doi.org/10.1016/j.jid.2020.02.026. Epub 2020 Mar 27. PMID: 32229141
4. Rundle CW, Hollingsworth P, Dellavalle RP. Artificial intelligence in dermatology. Clin Dermatol. 2021;39(4):657–66. https://doi.org/10.1016/j.clindermatol.2021.03.011. Epub 2021 Mar 19. PMID: 34809770

Role of Artificial Intelligence in Acne Vulgaris

2

Esraa Y. Salem and Esraa M. AlEdani

2.1 Introduction

Acne vulgaris, habitually called acne, is a chronic inflammatory condition of the sebaceous glands present on the skin. It affects all humans of any age, which may affect their psychological condition. The lesions may differ in appearance according to severity; they could be comedones, papules, pustules, nodules, cysts, or scars on the face, neck, and back. Acne is globally ranked as the eighth most common disease with a prevalence of 9.4%, and its incidence has been increasing lately. The underlying etiology has been attributed to multiple factors including diet, *C. acnes* (short for *Cutibacterium acnes*), also known as *P. acnes* (short for *Propionibacterium acnes*), and genetics.

The concern about late diagnosis and treatment, misdiagnosis, and high costs has been rising with the rise of incidence; hence the use of technology, artificial intelligence specifically, to deal with such concern is recommended. Artificial intelligence (AI) is a field of computer science that can mimic human intelligence through learning from data, thus giving precise analysis of complex data. The role of artificial intelligence (AI) has been rising in the diagnosis of dermatological diseases, drug designing, treatment, follow-up, and more.

E. Y. Salem (✉)
Modern University for Technology and Information, Cairo, Egypt
e-mail: esraa.92352@Medicine.mti.edu.eg

E. M. AlEdani
University of Basrah, College of Medicine, Basra, Iraq

E. M. AlEdani, H. I. Maibach (eds.), *Applications of Artificial Intelligence in Common Dermatological Diseases*, Updates in Clinical Dermatology,
https://doi.org/10.1007/978-3-031-78139-1_2

2.2 Finding Etiology

Metagenomic sequencing is a method of analysis of all genes of microbes in a given sample. This method can be used to identify the microbiota of the microorganisms contributing to acne vulgaris which can aid in prevention, diagnosis, and treatment. Wand and colleagues applied metagenomic sequencing to data of three different skin states: face skin of healthy people as normal control (NC), healthy face skin of acne patients (HS), and diseased face skin of acne patients (DS). The methods used to determine the most contributing lipids to each skin type were principal component analysis (PCA) and kernel principal component analysis (KPCA). Moreover, multisets of canonical correlation analysis (MCCA) method were implemented to retrieve lipids that can differentiate between three mentioned skin states. They found that the lipid of No. 1240 described as *PS (22: 6 (4Z, 7Z, 10Z, 13Z, 16Z, 19Z)/18: 1(9Z))* can be used to characterize DS sample set, lipids of No. 608 described as *PC (20: 0/26: 0)* and No. 2334 described as *GlcAbeta-Cer (d18: 1/18: 0)* can be used to characterize HS sample set, and lipids of No. 1264 described as *PS (22: 6 (4Z, 7Z, 10Z, 13Z, 16Z, 19Z)/19: 1(9Z))* and No. 1311 described as *PS (22: 6 (4Z, 7Z, 10Z, 13Z, 16Z, 19Z)/19: 0)* can be used to characterize NC sample set.

The study of genetics has been on the rise for they are essential factors in determining an individual's predisposition to diseases, one of which is acne vulgaris, as well as understanding their origins, acting as genetic markers, and facilitating personalized management. Driven by this idea, Chua et al. implemented Q-learning, a machine learning approach, to genetic data from three datasets extracted from the Gene Expression Omnibus (GEO) database, namely, GSE108110, GSE53795, and GSE6475. For the first dataset, the genes CD86 and AGPAT3 were biologically confirmed to be correlated to acne. For the second dataset, TMPRSS11D, DSG3, and TNFRSF1B genes were biologically confirmed to be correlated to acne, whereas, for the third dataset, PI3, C5AR1, and KRT16 genes were biologically confirmed to be correlated to acne.

2.3 Diagnosis

In dermatology, the role of artificial intelligence is becoming more and more significant. Computer vision is a type of artificial intelligence; as the name implies, it refers to how computers see visual input, such as images and movies (Fig. 2.1). Artificial intelligence (AI), more especially deep learning technology, and algorithms—most notably convolutional neural networks (CNN) (Fig. 2.2)—are two necessary components for computer vision to function. Furthermore, the use of computer-aided methods helps eliminate inter-rater and intra-rater variability, saves time and money, and is subjective. In this chapter, we will discuss the growing role of artificial intelligence in acne vulgaris.

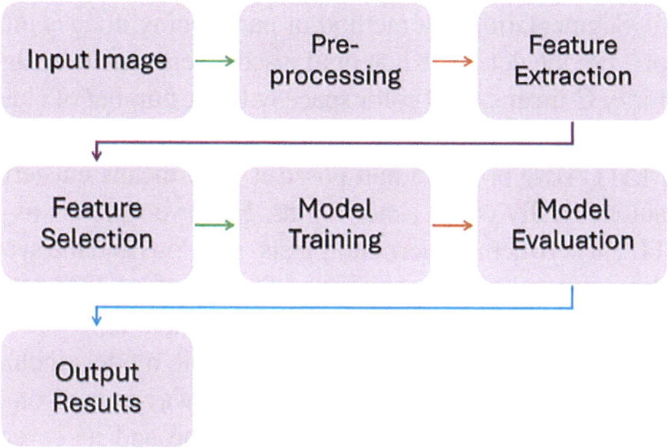

Fig. 2.1 Basic steps of computer vision

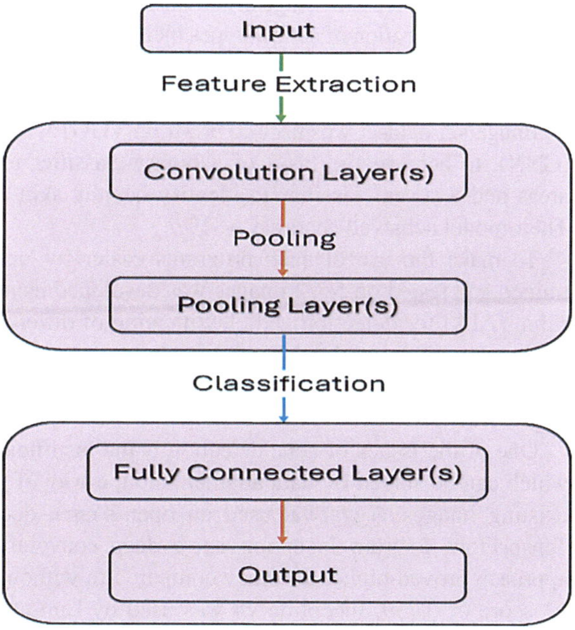

Fig. 2.2 Basic convolutional neural network (CNN) architecture

2.3.1 Detection and Classification

In 2012, Humayun and colleagues applied a template matching algorithm with chi-square correlation for localization of acne, matching the image features to features of a template. However, the algorithm had its limitations due to low-quality images, variable illumination, and rough skin texture which they proposed to overcome by pre-processing images with N-kernel. The proposed system showed an F1 score of 0.75. Image quality and illumination variability remained an issue; Seonguk et al. developed an acne image acquiring system that produced higher-quality images with shadow-free illumination, and images were then processed using MATLAB® program for lesion counting and showed a positive predictive value >70%.

Segmentation is a method of partitioning images into clusters to make it easier to process the details. Khan et al. used a segmentation algorithm with color spaces and fuzzy C-means. YIQ color space with the number of clusters equal to three showed the highest accuracy of 92.63%. Fajarnés et al. also used a segmentation algorithm run by MATLAB® program and based it on k-means clustering of fluorescence images to automatically count acne lesions. However, there was a maximum inconsistency of 11.2% between the dermatologists' opinions and the system, but regardless they claim their system's efficacy to be >90%. Another example of segmentation of k-means algorithm was also used by Nawar et al. and it proved its efficiency through an accuracy of 91.67%. An ensemble of multiple models including skin segmentation, body part detection, and acne identification was trained on an augmented version of the FSD dataset; its goal was to detect acne and its severity. A different segmentation method called region growing was used by Budhi and colleagues; this method showed high accuracy and easier usage in comparison to other segmentation methods in detection and classification of acne to types including papules, pustules, nodules, and cysts. They also tried self-organizing map, a type of artificial neural networks, which detected acne well, but wasn't as satisfactory in acne classification.

ImageNet dataset was used to pre-train VGG16, a convolutional neural network (CNN), to achieve the tasks of a binary-classifier to identify skin-and-non-skin areas and a seven-classifier to identify healthy skin and six acne vulgaris types. Their model achieved accuracy >81%.

To make the use of such programs easier for dermatologists, an application trained and tested on 5972 images was developed using artificial intelligence algorithm (AIA) for detection and classification of different acne lesions based on the GEA scale; the model achieved an average accuracy of 84%, 61%, and 72% for inflammatory, noninflammatory, and post-inflammatory hyperpigmentation lesions, respectively.

One of the issues of acne detection is the insufficiency of high-quality images, which can be solved by data augmentation, a way of generating new images from existing images. Aggarwal used an open-source deep learning approach called TensorFlow, to train Inception v3, a deep convolutional neural network. Their approach proved higher accuracy compared to without data augmentation, with an F1 score of 0.759. Inception v4 was used by Lim et al. to detect and grade acne based on the IGA scale; higher accuracy was directly proportional to increasing image resolution; a 1200 × 1600 resolution cultivated an accuracy of 67%. Inception v4 was also used in another study to predict differential diagnoses for multiple dermatological conditions; on the top of the list was acne with an accuracy of 66%. Yang et al. used a pre-trained Inception v3 on ImageNet dataset, as well as an image augmentation technique, ImageDataGenerator, in Keras. The average precision of their proposed method was 80%. Pancholi et al. investigated multiple pre-trained deep learning algorithms with classification methods. Inception v3 with logistic regression was 99.5% accurate. Inception v3 was also used in another study and achieved a 0.32 precision for acne.

The use of CNN has been on the rise. Junayed and colleagues proposed AcneNet, a model based on deep residual neural network, which is a type of CNN, using TensorFlow and Keras in the backend and trained on images from *dermanet.com*.

TensorFlow and Keras are open-source libraries for deep learning. The AcneNet model showed promising results for detecting and classifying acne into different types with an accuracy >90% for all classes. In 2022, Junayed and colleagues proposed a new model to better the performance of AcneNet by using a dual encoder made of a CNN and a transformer for image segmentation, which resulted in 88.1% accuracy. Similarly, Tibot is an AI application based on CNN for the detection of different dermatological conditions including acne for which it showed a predictive accuracy of 84% as observed in a study conducted in 2020, which evolved to 91.7% in another study in 2023; however, there is a limitation of unstandardized images in terms of focus, illumination, angle, and lack of users' knowledge about skin types. Further use of CNN algorithms has been witnessed. Zhu et al. used modified EfficientNet-b4 CNN algorithm, for the classification of multiple skin diseases including acne. Their approach achieved an average accuracy of 92.75%.

In 2021, Min et al. propose ACNet based on augmented images of acne lesions from ImageNet and ACNE04 datasets with the implementation of ResNet101 algorithm which proved to have a mean average precision (mAP) of 81.8. Biloborodova et al. augmented data from ACNE04 dataset and implemented it in ResNet152, a CNN model. Their model achieved an accuracy of 85%. Zhang and scientists used the same dataset, ACNE04; however they used ResNet50 and YOLOv5 algorithms for detection and severity classification, respectively. However, a limitation of their proposed method is decreased effectiveness with increased acne density. Huynh and researchers proposed a model composed of an acne object detection algorithm, Faster R-CNN, with a ResNet50 backbone achieving a mean average precision (mAP) of 0.54 and a severity grading algorithm called LightGBM achieving 85% accuracy; however the model faced difficulty learning to recognize scars. The infamous ACNE04 dataset was used again but this time it shows low quality; the images were used to develop a publicly available mobile application to assess the presence and extent of acne using Faster R-CNN and ResNet101 algorithms to achieve a mAP of 0.536. Nevertheless, there were some limitations including difficulty detecting small objects and confusion with other similar skin conditions. AcneGrader is an ensemble model used for assessing severity of acne; it is composed of 10 ResNet18 in combination with 20 ResNet34 and a pruning model retrieving a 93.18% accuracy. ResNet50 was used also by Li et al. and harvested an average precision of 0.507; their study is characterized by detailed classification of acne into eight types of inconsistency. Kiran et al. used Inception-ResNet50 and MobileNet models for detection of acne and dark circles obtaining a 99% accuracy. Yadav and scientists also used ResNet18 to a custom dataset Kaggle dataset that only included fair skin imageries, which help achieve a better accuracy of up to 90%.

A deep neural network model called OpenCV was integrated in a study by Malgina and colleagues in the form of a smartphone application for easy utilization. The application exhibited an accuracy of 83% assessing facial acne severity and type. Naidu et al. developed Dermato, which also used OpenCV with Inception v3 trained on Keras optimizer to categorize acne images into four types (comedones, papules, pustules, and rosacea) and then into four levels (0–3); compared with other algorithms like VGG16, Xception, and Fastai, Inception v3 retrieved the highest accuracy of 89.39%.

AlexNet is an advanced CNN architecture. AlexNet was used to identify and classify different skin diseases including acne vulgaris. The images for training were obtained from DermNet, to harvest an accuracy of 85.7% for acne identification. Bokefode and Shinde compared three different models, and their comparison showed CNN to have the highest accuracy of 96.59%. EfficientNet is another deep CNN model that was used by Prodeep et al. to detect acne and rosacea; their model results in 99.74% accuracy. Furthermore, Quattrini et al. applied an ensemble model consisting of VGG-1, DenseNet121 on ImageNet dataset images showing an average precision of 59.89%. As is noticeable, personal images are being used for the recognition of skin diseases such as acne vulgaris; as the image sharing increases, the need for confidentiality rises as well. Hence, Hossen et al. used a federated learning approach along with the CNN model. The CNN model achieved an 86% precision and the federated learning approach an accuracy of 94.15%. In another study, a system using both VGG16 and EfficientNet (B3) was used to retrieve an accuracy of 69% in detection of multiple dermatological conditions.

A hybrid system composed of CNNs, recurrent neural networks (RNNs), and a long short-term memory (LSTM) has shown better performance in detection of multiple skin conditions including but not limited to acne, eczema, and melanoma. In hopes of resolving the existing issue of cloudy boundaries and small sizes of acne, Zhang et al. constructed a novel dataset named AcneSCU, composed of 276 high-resolution facial images, with precise annotations. They also proposed a new Spatial Aware Region Proposal Network (SA-RPN) for acne detection. RPN and SA-RPN have similar functions. The distinction is that SA-RPN uses two different types of convolution layers to separate the representation learning for the original RPN's classification and localization. Their system proposed an average precision of 0.268.

Attention Enhanced Feature Pyramid Network (AEFPN) is an extractor of image features of object detection characterized by accurate and fast performance; it was used in combination with YOLOX-S, MixAug for augmentation, and SimOTA tiny; and the performance was assessed with AP50 achieving 0.6319. A study was conducted on 1,156,703 facial images in 2024 in China to detect subtypes and the trend inconsistency of acne among adult females in China using an ensemble system made of ResNet50, Feature Pyramid Network (FPN) module, and Region Proposal Network (RPN).

In a study by Navaro and scientists, they implemented Speed-Up Robust Features (SURF) algorithm, k-means clustering, and support vector machine (SVM) in a Bag of Feature algorithm showing an accuracy of 96%. Kumar et al. used a CNN-SVM model achieving a high accuracy of 97% for acne vulgaris classification.

YOLO (You Only Look Once) is a single-stage object detection tool that uses CNN algorithms, compared to other CNN algorithms. YOLO is considered better than other CNN algorithms due to its higher performance without compromising accuracy. The YOLO model has had multiple improvements and has been implemented multiple times for the detection of acne vulgaris, as YOLOv3 in one study and YOLOv5 in another study, and obtained a mAP of 0.834. Kahatapitiya and researchers even used CNN in developing an AI-based dermoscope, which is basically a microscope for the skin to detect different conditions; YOLOv8 and R-CNN were used for this goal and retrieved an 84.9% precision. PP-YOLO is a modified YOLOv3 model based on PaddlePaddle, a deep learning framework trained on 1213 facial images with different acne lesions to achieve a mAP of 28.48; the tool was evaluated by 8 dermatology professionals for identifying 5 subtypes of acne lesions and for categorizing lesions into inflammatory and non-inflammatory.

2.3.2 Detection of Complications

Acne vulgaris can heal with scars in 95% of patients; despite the high prevalence, sometimes, it is misdiagnosed due to the different types requiring different treatments; hence, Junayed et al. proposed ScarNet, a program for acne scar detection and classification; the program was trained and tested with a dataset named "5-class Acne Scar" that the scientists proposed in their work; it contained 250 images. The five classes labeled in the dataset are hypertrophic, keloidal, icepick, rolling scars, and boxcar. Hypertrophic and keloid scars are both caused by collagen deposition leading to raised skin; they differ in extent with the former being within and the latter being beyond the borders of the original lesion. Icepick scars are v-shaped, deep, and narrow as if caused by an icepick. Rolling scars have gently slopped edges, while boxcar scars are round or oval with flat floors. The images from the dataset were preprocessed and augmented and fed into a deep convolutional neural network (CNN) retrieving a 92.35% accuracy.

2.4 Teledermatology

AcneCheck is a teledermatology service website built based on application programing interface (API) for detection and grading of acne vulgaris. The website was assessed by the telehealth usability questionnaire (TUQ) assessing usefulness, utility and learnability, user interface quality, interaction quality, reliability, satisfaction, and future use to achieve an average score of 5.92. They went a further step and added a video conferencing feature with a dermatologist and the ability to schedule appointments.

2.5 Treatment Options

Antimicrobial resistance in *Cutibacterium acnes (C. acnes)* has been on the rise, leading to the need to discover an alternative. Antimicrobial peptides (AMPs) are naturally existing proteins as part of innate immunity response; they are proposed as an alternative treatment for *C. acnes*, and for time efficiency artificial intelligence has been used to design new *C. acnes*-associated AMPs; they also inhibited *E. coli*, *S. aureus*, and *C. albicans*. Furthermore, all evaluated AMPs exhibit minimal hemolytic and cytotoxic effects.

Another solution to the antimicrobial resistance, a replacement to the side effect of retinoids, and a way of distant healthcare monitoring is the smart low-level laser therapy (LLLT) system developed to diagnose and treat skin diseases including acne; it is anti-inflammatory, antimicrobial, skin rejuvenating, and a safe noninvasive alternative. However, it's recommended that its clinical application be explored more.

In fear of self-misdiagnosis and self-prescription, a fuzzy knowledge-based system was developed to diagnose and grade acne and recommend appropriate treatment with appropriate dosages. Even worse, displeasure with acne consequences including pores and scars can encourage patients to self-medicate with skincare products that might irritate and deteriorate the skin, which motivated Lin et al. to design a system deploying deep residual neural networks for diagnosing, grading, and recommending facial skincare products.

2.6 Follow-Up

The methods used for detection and classification of acne lesions can also be used for follow-up of patients. For instance, segmentation was used to predict the time required for full recovery after treatment and OpenCV was utilized to evaluate the efficacy of the treatment used.

2.7 ChatGPT as a Clinical Guide

Since the release of ChatGPT, a form of generative AI, it has been a hot topic and a handy tool for a lot of users, some of which are acne patients who wonder about their condition, what caused it, and how to treat it. A group of researchers decided to investigate whether this tool was reliable; using the ChatGPT 3.5 model, they found that 66% of the responses were right but insufficient and 34% were comprehensive; however, the responses for acne management was 56% accurate (relatively low), suggesting that ChatGPT falls short of giving treatment recommendations for acne vulgaris. Successive advanced ChatGPT models may show varying results.

2.8 Conclusion

In this chapter, a review of literature has shown the critical role played by artificial intelligence (AI) in a globally common skin condition like acne vulgaris, commonly known as acne. It has an emerging role in detecting the etiology through genetic sequencing of the microbiota and the most correlated lipids to each type. Moreover, it has proven useful in lessening the variability between dermatologists in diagnosis of acne lesions and scars, saving time for both the patient and the clinical personnel and expenses, as well as connecting patients to professionals when needed with remote means. However, the role of dermatologists can't be omitted, and it is always safe to visit a professional in suspicious conditions. Furthermore, AI has shown advances in the management sector as it has been used to develop personalized drugs for better efficiency and less side effects, in addition to predicting the need for treatment and recommending options for each stage of acne and following up the recovery process. Finally, despite ChatGPT's high performance, researchers still hold doubt about its reliability in answering acne-related questions asked by patients, especially regarding treatment.

References

1. Chua YC, Nies HW, Kamsani II, Hashim H, Yusoff Y, Chan WH, et al. Ai-driven Q-learning for personalized acne genetics: innovative approaches and potential genetic markers. Egypt Info J. 2024;26:100484. https://doi.org/10.1016/j.eij.2024.100484.
2. Junayed MS, Islam MB, Jeny AA, Sadeghzadeh A, Biswas T, Shah AF. ScarNet: development and validation of a novel deep CNN model for acne scar classification with a new dataset. IEEE Access [Internet]. 2022;10:1245–58. https://doi.org/10.1109/ACCESS.2021.3138021.
3. Tan JKL, Bhate K. A global perspective on the epidemiology of acne. Br J Dermatol. 2015;172:3–12. https://doi.org/10.1111/bjd.13462.
4. Phan DT, Ta QB, Ly CD, Nguyen CH, Park S, Choi J, et al. Smart low level laser therapy system for automatic facial dermatological disorder diagnosis. IEEE J Biomed Health Inform. 2023;27(3):1546–57. https://doi.org/10.1109/jbhi.2023.3237875.
5. Charulatha G, Dineskkumar R, Kaleeswari B, Lakshmipriya K. Computer-aided design for skin disease identification and categorization using image processing. J Sci Comput Eng Res. 2023;6(4):24–8. https://doi.org/10.46379/jscer.2023.060407.
6. Marri SS, Inamadar AC, Janagond AB, Albadri W. Analyzing the predictability of an Artificial Intelligence App (Tibot) in the diagnosis of dermatological conditions: a cross-sectional study. JMIR Dermatology. 2023:6. https://doi.org/10.2196/45529.
7. De A, Sarda A, Gupta S, Das S. Use of artificial intelligence in dermatology. Indian J Dermatol. 2020;65(5):352. https://doi.org/10.4103/ijd.ijd_418_20.
8. Wang Y, Sun M, Duan Y. Metagenomic sequencing analysis for acne using machine learning methods adapted to single or multiple data. Comput Math Methods Med. 2021:1–11. https://doi.org/10.1155/2021/8008731.
9. Young AT, Xiong M, Pfau J, Keiser MJ, Wei ML. Artificial intelligence in dermatology: a primer. J Invest Dermatol. 2020;140(8):1504–12. https://doi.org/10.1016/j.jid.2020.02.026.
10. Zhang H, Ma T. Acne detection by ensemble neural networks. Sensors. 2022;22(18):6828. https://doi.org/10.3390/s22186828.
11. Shen X, Zhang J, Yan C, Zhou H. An automatic diagnosis method of facial acne vulgaris based on convolutional neural network. Sci Rep. 2018;8(1) https://doi.org/10.1038/s41598-018-24204-6.
12. Bokefode K, Shinde S. Skin disease diagnosis by using different machine learning & deep learning approach. 6th International Conference on Computing, Communication, Control and Automation (ICCUBEA); 2022. https://doi.org/10.1109/iccubea54992.2022.10010801
13. Humayun J, Malik AS, Belhaouari SB, Kamel N, Yap FB. Localization of acne lesion through template matching. 4th International Conference on Intelligent and Advanced Systems (ICIAS2012); 2012. https://doi.org/10.1109/icias.2012.6306166
14. Min S, Kong H, Yoon C, Kim HC, Suh DH. Development and evaluation of an automatic acne lesion detection program using digital image processing. Skin Res Technol. 2012;19(1) https://doi.org/10.1111/j.1600-0846.2012.00660.x.
15. Khan J, Malik AS, Kamel N, Dass SC, Affandi AM. Segmentation of acne lesion using fuzzy C-means technique with intelligent selection of the desired cluster. 37th Annual International

Conference of the IEEE Engineering in Medicine and Biology Society (EMBC); 2015. https://doi.org/10.1109/embc.2015.7319042
16. Peris Fajarnés G, Moncho Santonja M, Defez García B, Lengua I. Segmentation methods for acne vulgaris images: proposal of a new methodology applied to fluorescence images. Skin Res Technol. 2020;26(5):734–9. https://doi.org/10.1111/srt.12865.
17. Nawar A, Sabuz NK, Siddiquee SMT, Rabbani M, Biswas AA, Majumder A. Skin disease recognition: a machine vision based approach. 7th International Conference on Advanced Computing and Communication Systems (ICACCS); 2021. https://doi.org/10.1109/icaccs51430.2021.9441980
18. Maroni G, Ermidoro M, Previdi F, Bigini G. Automated detection, extraction and counting of acne lesions for automatic evaluation and tracking of acne severity. IEEE Symposium Series on Computational Intelligence (SSCI); 2017. https://doi.org/10.1109/ssci.2017.8280925
19. Budhi GS, Adipranata R, Gunawan A. Acne segmentation and classification using region growing and self-organizing map. International Conference on Soft Computing, Intelligent System and Information Technology (ICSIIT); 2017. https://doi.org/10.1109/icsiit.2017.62
20. Seité S, Khammari A, Benzaquen M, Moyal D, Dréno B. Development and accuracy of an artificial intelligence algorithm for acne grading from smartphone photographs. Exp Dermatol. 2019;28(11):1252–7. https://doi.org/10.1111/exd.14022.
21. Seite S, Moyal D, Abidi K, Le Dantec G, Khammari A, Benzaquen M, et al. Development and accuracy of an artificial intelligence algorithm for acne evaluation. J Am Acad Dermatol. 2020;83(6) https://doi.org/10.1016/j.jaad.2020.06.156.
22. Aggarwal LP. Data augmentation in dermatology image recognition using machine learning. Skin Res Technol. 2019;25(6):815–20. https://doi.org/10.1111/srt.12726.
23. Lim ZV, Akram F, Ngo CP, Winarto AA, Lee WQ, Liang K, et al. Automated grading of acne vulgaris by deep learning with convolutional neural networks. Skin Res Technol. 2019;26(2):187–92. https://doi.org/10.1111/srt.12794.
24. Liu Y, Jain A, Eng C, Way DH, Lee K, Bui P, et al. A deep learning system for differential diagnosis of skin diseases. Nat Med. 2020;26(6):900–8. https://doi.org/10.1038/s41591-020-0842-3.
25. Yang Y, Guo L, Wu Q, Zhang M, Zeng R, Ding H, et al. Construction and evaluation of a deep learning model for assessing acne vulgaris using clinical images. Dermatol Ther. 2021;11(4):1239–48. https://doi.org/10.1007/s13555-021-00541-9.
26. Pancholi N, Goel S, Nijhawan R, Gupta S. Classification and detection of acne on the skin using deep learning algorithms. 19th OITS International Conference on Information Technology (OCIT); 2021. https://doi.org/10.1109/ocit53463.2021.00032
27. Shetty SB, Nishith, Kamath CS, Nishani. Skin disease classification using InceptionV3 model. International Conference on Artificial Intelligence and Data Engineering (AIDE); 2022. https://doi.org/10.1109/aide57180.2022.10059678
28. Junayed MS, Jeny AA, Atik ST, Neehal N, Karim A, Azam S, et al. AcneNet - a deep CNN based classification approach for acne classes. 12th International Conference on Information & Communication Technology and System (ICTS); 2019. 10.1109/icts.2019.8850935
29. Junayed MS, Islam MB, Anjum N. A transformer-based versatile network for acne vulgaris segmentation. Innovations in Intelligent Systems and Applications Conference (ASYU); 2022. https://doi.org/10.1109/asyu56188.2022.9925323
30. Patil A, Patil S, Rao D, Basar F, Bate S. Assessment of Tibot® artificial intelligence application in prediction of diagnosis in dermatological conditions: results of a single centre study. Indian Dermatol Online J. 2020;11(6):910. https://doi.org/10.4103/idoj.idoj_61_20.
31. Zhu C-Y, Wang Y-K, Chen H-P, Gao K-L, Shu C, Wang J-C, et al. A deep learning based framework for diagnosing multiple skin diseases in a clinical environment. Front Med. 2021:8. https://doi.org/10.3389/fmed.2021.626369.
32. Min K, Lee G-H, Lee S-W. ACNet: mask-aware attention with dynamic context enhancement for robust acne detection. IEEE International Conference on Systems, Man, and Cybernetics (SMC); 2021. https://doi.org/10.1109/smc52423.2021.9659243

33. Biloborodova T, Skarga-Bandurova I, Koverha M, Skarha-Bandurov I, Yevsieieva Y. A learning framework for medical image-based intelligent diagnosis from imbalanced datasets. Stud Health Technol Inform. 2021; https://doi.org/10.3233/shti210801.
34. Huynh QT, Nguyen PH, Le HX, Ngo LT, Trinh N-T, Tran MT-T, et al. Automatic acne object detection and acne severity grading using smartphone images and artificial intelligence. Diagnostics. 2022;12(8):1879. https://doi.org/10.3390/diagnostics12081879.
35. Wen H, Yu W, Wu Y, Zhao J, Liu X, Kuang Z, et al. Acne detection and severity evaluation with interpretable convolutional neural network models. Technol Health Care. 2022;30:143–53. https://doi.org/10.3233/thc-228014.
36. Liu S, Fan Y, Duan M, Wang Y, Su G, Ren Y, et al. AcneGrader: an ensemble pruning of the deep learning base models to grade acne. Skin Res Technol. 2022;28(5):677–88. https://doi.org/10.1111/srt.13166.
37. Li J, Du D, Zhang J, Liu W, Wang J, Wei X, et al. Development and validation of an artificial intelligence-powered acne grading system incorporating lesion identification. Front Med. 2023:10. https://doi.org/10.3389/fmed.2023.1255704.
38. Kiran MK, Meda Ravi K, Umadevi V. Facial skin analysis for detection of dark circles and acne. Third International Conference on Artificial Intelligence and Smart Energy (ICAIS); 2023. https://doi.org/10.1109/icais56108.2023.10073775
39. Yadav R, Jain A, Sharma S. Acne detection care system using deep learning. 11th International Conference on Reliability, Infocom Technologies and Optimization (Trends and Future Directions) (ICRITO); 2024. https://doi.org/10.1109/icrito61523.2024.10522412
40. Malgina E, Kurochkina M-A. Development of the mobile application for assessing facial acne severity from photos. IEEE Conference of Russian Young Researchers in Electrical and Electronic Engineering (ElConRus); 2021. https://doi.org/10.1109/elconrus51938.2021.9396382.
41. Naidu K, Kareppa O, Menon S, Bhole C, Poojary S. Dermato: a deep learning based application for acne subtype and severity detection. International Conference on Innovative Data Communication Technologies and Application (ICIDCA); 2023. https://doi.org/10.1109/icidca56705.2023.10100165
42. Shanthi T, Sabeenian RS, Anand R. Automatic diagnosis of skin diseases using convolution neural network. Microprocess Microsyst. 2020;76:103074. https://doi.org/10.1016/j.micpro.2020.103074.
43. Prodeep AR, Araf R, Ray P, Ulubbi MdS, Ananna SN, Mridha MF. Acne and Rosacea detection from images using deep CNN's Efficientnet. International Conference on Advances in Computing, Communication and Applied Informatics (ACCAI); 2022. https://doi.org/10.1109/accai53970.2022.9752534
44. Quattrini A, Boër C, Leidi T, Paydar R. A deep learning-based facial acne classification system. Clin Cosmet Investig Dermatol. 2022;15:851–7. https://doi.org/10.2147/ccid.s360450.
45. Hossen MDN, Panneerselvam V, Koundal D, Ahmed K, Bui FM, Ibrahim SM. Federated machine learning for detection of skin diseases and enhancement of internet of medical things (IOMT) security. IEEE J Biomed Health Inform. 2023;27(2):835–41. https://doi.org/10.1109/jbhi.2022.3149288.
46. Ghadekar P, Bongulwar A, Jadhav A, Ahire R, Dumbre A, Ali S. Ensemble approach to solve multiple skin disease classification using deep learning. International Conference on Device Intelligence, Computing and Communication Technologies, (DICCT); 2023. https://doi.org/10.1109/dicct56244.2023.10110278
47. Varalakshmi K, Revathi A. Computer-aided design for skin disease identification and categorization using deep learning. Seventh International Conference on Image Information Processing (ICIIP); 2023. https://doi.org/10.1109/iciip61524.2023.10537681
48. Zhang J, Zhang L, Wang J, Wei X, Li J, Jiang X, et al. SA-RPN: a spacial aware region proposal network for acne detection. IEEE J Biomed Health Inform. 2023;27(11):5439–48. https://doi.org/10.1109/jbhi.2023.3304727.
49. Ma X, Lu J, Liu X, Kuang H. An acne detector for skin image based on attention enhanced feature pyramid networks. IEEE 3rd International Conference on Information Technology, Big Data and Artificial Intelligence (ICIBA); 2023. https://doi.org/10.1109/iciba56860.2023.10165620

50. Li T, Ma X, Li Z, Yu N, Song J, Ma Z, et al. Facial adult female acne in China: an analysis based on artificial intelligence over one million. Skin Res Technol. 2024;30(4) https://doi.org/10.1111/srt.13693.
51. Navarro MaC, Bustillos E, Barfeh DP. Skin disease analysis using digital image processing. International Conference on Computational Intelligence and Knowledge Economy (ICCIKE); 2019. https://doi.org/10.1109/iccike47802.2019.9004267
52. Kumar V, Banerjee D, Chauhan R, Kukreti S, Gill KS. Optimizing skin disease classification: a comprehensive investigation of CNN-SVM hybrid models with layer configurations. 3rd International Conference for Innovation in Technology (INOCON); 2024. https://doi.org/10.1109/inocon60754.2024.10511340
53. Nivedita V, Subramaniam K, Ramya M, Parameshachari BD. Machine learning based skin disease analyzer with image processing. IEEE North Karnataka Subsection Flagship International Conference (NKCon); 2022. https://doi.org/10.1109/nkcon56289.2022.10127040
54. Wu Z, Lai G, Lin X, Chung KL. A real-time skin disease recognition system based on YOLOv5 algorithm. IEEE 6th International Conference on Electronic Information and Communication Technology (ICEICT); 2023. https://doi.org/10.1109/iceict57916.2023.10245878
55. Kahatapitiya NS, Wijethunge A, Edirisinghe S, Silva BN, Jeon M, Kim J, et al. Development of convolutional neural network-based AI-dermatoscope for non-invasive skin assessments. 5th International Conference on Advancements in Computing (ICAC); 2023. https://doi.org/10.1109/icac60630.2023.10417424
56. Kim DH, Sun S, Cho SI, Kong H-J, Lee JW, Lee JH, et al. Automated facial acne lesion detecting and counting algorithm for acne severity evaluation and its utility in assisting dermatologists. Am J Clin Dermatol. 2023;24(4):649–59. https://doi.org/10.1007/s40257-023-00777-5.
57. Samonte MJ, Borja J, Delariarte LM, Ebanen JA. AcneCheck: an acne severity grading in teledermatology through computer vision. 13th International Conference on Software Technology and Engineering (ICSTE); 2023. https://doi.org/10.1109/icste61649.2023.00027
58. Dong Q, Wang S, Miao Y, Luo H, Weng Z, Yu L. Novel antimicrobial peptides against Cutibacterium acnes designed by deep learning. Sci Rep. 2024;14(1) https://doi.org/10.1038/s41598-024-55205-3.
59. Phan DT, Ta QB, Huynh TC, Vo TH, Nguyen CH, Park S, et al. A smart led therapy device with an automatic facial acne vulgaris diagnosis based on deep learning and internet of things application. Comput Biol Med. 2021;136:104610. https://doi.org/10.1016/j.compbiomed.2021.104610.
60. Norizad PN, Mahmud Y, Noh NM, Abdul-Rahman S. Acne treatment recommender fuzzy knowledge-based system with image processing. 3rd International Conference on Artificial Intelligence and Data Sciences (AiDAS); 2022. https://doi.org/10.1109/aidas56890.2022.9918735
61. Lin T-Y, Chan H-T, Hsia C-H, Lai C-F. Facial skincare products' recommendation with computer vision technologies. Electronics. 2022;11(1):143. https://doi.org/10.3390/electronics11010143.
62. Lakdawala N, Channa L, Gronbeck C, Lakdawala N, Weston G, Sloan B, et al. Assessing the accuracy and comprehensiveness of ChatGPT in offering clinical guidance for atopic dermatitis and acne vulgaris. JMIR Dermatol. 2023;6 https://doi.org/10.2196/50409.

The Role of Artificial Intelligence in Psoriasis

3

N. L. Swathi, Syed Muhammad, Muhammad Muzzamil, Akhil Arun, H. Athul, and Esraa M. AlEdani

3.1 Introduction

3.1.1 The Burden of Psoriasis

The burden of psoriasis is multifaceted, encompassing not only the physical manifestations but also significant psychosocial and economic impacts. Psoriasis affects approximately 2–5% of the global population, with a higher prevalence observed in adults compared to children. This chronic inflammatory skin disorder is characterized by hyperproliferation of keratinocytes and an aberrant immune response involving cytokines such as TNF-α, IL-17, and IL-23.

N. L. Swathi (✉)
Department of Pharmacy Practice, Jawaharlal Nehru Technological University, Anantapur, India

S. Muhammad
Department of Clinical Pharmacy, Farooqia College of Pharmacy, Mysuru, India

M. Muzzamil
Department of Public Health, Health Services Academy, Islamabad, Pakistan

A. Arun
Department of Pharmacy Practice, Amrita School of Pharmacy, Amrita Vishwa Vidyapeetham, Aims Health Sciences Campus, Kochi, Kerala, India

H. Athul
Department of Pharmacy Practice, Nazareth College of Pharmacy, Thiruvalla, Kerala, India

E. M. AlEdani
University of Basrah, College of Medicine, Basra, Iraq

E. M. AlEdani, H. I. Maibach (eds.), *Applications of Artificial Intelligence in Common Dermatological Diseases*, Updates in Clinical Dermatology,
https://doi.org/10.1007/978-3-031-78139-1_3

3.1.1.1 Clinical Manifestations and Comorbidities

Psoriasis presents with various phenotypes including plaque psoriasis, guttate psoriasis, inverse psoriasis, pustular psoriasis, and erythrodermic psoriasis. Plaque psoriasis is the most common form, affecting about 80–90% of patients. Pustular psoriasis, although rare, poses significant clinical challenges due to its severe systemic involvement. Psoriatic arthritis (PsA) occurs in up to 30% of patients with psoriasis and is associated with substantial morbidity due to joint damage if not diagnosed early.

Comorbid conditions are prevalent among individuals with psoriasis. Metabolic syndrome components such as obesity, hypertension, dyslipidemia, and diabetes mellitus are significantly more common in psoriatic patients compared to the general population. Cardiovascular diseases are also a major concern due to chronic systemic inflammation. Additionally, mental health disorders including depression and anxiety are frequently reported among psoriatic patients due to the visible nature of the disease and its impact on quality of life.

3.1.1.2 Treatment Modalities

Management strategies for psoriasis have evolved significantly over recent years. Traditional therapies include topical agents like corticosteroids and vitamin D analogues for mild cases. Systemic treatments such as methotrexate, cyclosporine, and acitretin are reserved for moderate-to-severe cases or those unresponsive to topical treatments. Phototherapy remains a viable option for many patients.

Biologic therapies targeting specific immune pathways have revolutionized the treatment landscape for moderate-to-severe psoriasis. TNF inhibitors (e.g., adalimumab), IL-17 inhibitors (e.g., secukinumab), IL-12/23 inhibitors (e.g., ustekinumab), and IL-23 inhibitors (e.g., guselkumab) have shown superior efficacy compared to traditional systemic agents. However, biologics come with high costs and potential adverse effects including increased risk of infections.

Emerging therapies targeting novel pathways such as JAK inhibitors show promise in managing refractory cases but require further validation through large-scale clinical trials. Combination therapies involving biologics with conventional agents like methotrexate may enhance treatment efficacy while minimizing adverse effects.

3.1.1.3 Challenges in Management

Despite advancements in therapeutic options, several challenges persist in managing psoriasis effectively. Treatment resistance remains a significant issue; variability in patient response necessitates personalized treatment approaches guided by biomarkers and multi-omics technologies. Adverse effects associated with long-term use of systemic agents pose additional hurdles.

Economic burden is another critical aspect; direct costs include medications and healthcare visits, while indirect costs encompass lost productivity due to disability or absenteeism from work. A study highlighted that annual healthcare costs per patient can range from $11,000 to $13,000 depending on disease severity.

3.1.1.4 Special Populations

Paediatric psoriasis presents unique challenges due to differences in clinical presentation and limited approved treatment options. Children often exhibit smaller plaques with finer scales compared to adults; however severe forms can lead to significant psychosocial distress impacting their development. Similarly elderly patients may face complications related to comorbidities necessitating careful selection of therapeutic regimens considering potential drug interactions.

The burden of psoriasis extends beyond skin involvement, encompassing significant physical comorbidities and profound psychosocial impacts across all age groups, negatively affecting quality-of-life metrics. While biologic therapies offer promising outcomes, particularly for moderate-to-severe cases, their high cost and potential adverse effects necessitate careful, individualized use. This can be optimized through biomarker-driven personalized medicine approaches, ensuring tailored treatment strategies. For special populations, achieving a balance between efficacy and safety is crucial, requiring a holistic approach to comprehensive disease management. Future research should focus on elucidating the underlying pathophysiological mechanisms and developing innovative, targeted therapeutics to advance the field, ultimately improving patient outcomes on a global scale.

3.1.2 Challenges in Psoriasis Diagnosis and Management

Diagnosing psoriasis, especially its nail involvement and PsA, remains a formidable task due to overlapping symptoms with other dermatological and rheumatological conditions. Nail psoriasis affects up to 80% of patients with psoriatic lesions, presenting as pitting, leukonychia, red lunula, onycholysis, oil spots, and subungual hyperkeratosis. The Nail Psoriasis Severity Index (NAPSI) is commonly used for assessment but lacks specificity in distinguishing between nail psoriasis and other nail disorders such as lichen planus.

The diagnosis of PsA further complicates the clinical picture. Up to one-third of psoriasis patients develop PsA, which can manifest with peripheral arthritis, dactylitis, enthesitis, axial disease, and nail involvement. Early diagnosis is crucial to prevent irreversible joint damage; however, it often mimics other inflammatory arthritides like rheumatoid arthritis or gout. Screening tools such as musculoskeletal ultrasound have been suggested for early detection but require further validation.

3.1.3 Pathophysiology Overview

The pathophysiology of psoriasis involves a complex interplay between genetic predisposition and immune-mediated mechanisms. HLA-Cw6 is one of the most strongly associated alleles with psoriasis susceptibility. It influences disease onset, severity, phenotypic features like guttate psoriasis, and treatment responses. Patients carrying HLA-Cw6 are more responsive to methotrexate and ustekinumab but less so to conventional therapies in high-need cases.

Cytokines play a pivotal role in the inflammatory cascade characteristic of psoriasis. IL-23/Th17 axis has been identified as central to its pathogenesis. Biologics targeting IL-23p19 subunit like guselkumab have shown efficacy in preventing progression from skin psoriasis to PsA by reducing synovio-entheseal inflammation. Tildrakizumab also targets IL-23p19 and has demonstrated significant improvement in Psoriasis Area and Severity Index (PASI) scores with sustained efficacy over 2 years.

Nail involvement adds another layer of complexity due to its refractory nature. The same cytokines implicated in skin lesions are involved in nail pathology; however, treatment responses vary significantly. Topical therapies suffice for mild cases, while biologics are reserved for severe or refractory cases. Emerging treatments like JAK inhibitors show promise but require more extensive studies for validation.

3.1.3.1 Comorbidities

Psoriasis is frequently associated with comorbid conditions such as metabolic syndrome and non-alcoholic fatty liver disease (NAFLD). Chronic inflammation underpins both conditions through mechanisms involving insulin resistance and systemic inflammation markers like TNF-alpha. Managing these comorbidities necessitates a holistic approach encompassing lifestyle modifications alongside pharmacotherapy.

Dietary interventions have shown potential benefits; weight reduction through hypocaloric diets significantly improves disease severity in overweight patients with psoriasis or PsA. Vitamin D supplementation is weakly recommended for PsA patients based on low-quality data but may offer adjunctive benefits when combined with standard therapies.

3.2 Applications of AI in Psoriasis

The incorporation of artificial intelligence (AI) technologies could greatly benefit even a common chronic inflammatory condition like psoriasis. AI could be used for the early diagnosis and risk management domain. Lesion detection is also used as a major example of how automated image analysis for this purpose can be implemented, further demonstrating the technology potential to adapt commonly available AI tools (Gomolin et al. 2020), for one-off use in hepatology. This could be achieved by using AI-based analysis of patient record data [36] to predict the time-to-event model of psoriasis onset facilitating the development and implementation of early preventive strategies and personalized care planning.

Moving forwards, phenotyping and subtyping of psoriasis as suggested by Barlow (2023) indicate a positive shift towards utilizing AI models in common inflammatory diseases like psoriasis. Machine learning algorithms, as highlighted by Lunge et al. [56], can help in predicting treatment responses and tailoring therapies to individual patients, optimizing outcomes. Additionally, for clinicians Deisms et al. (2023) proposed that AI can assist in their decision support systems which can enhance treatment decision-making processes, ensuring more precise and effective care delivery.

In the domain of monitoring of psoriasis, the integration of wearable devices and AI for disease activity tracking, as discussed by Reinders (2023), presents a novel approach to continuous monitoring and management. AI-based analysis of imaging data, as highlighted by Huang et al. [12, 34], can offer insights into treatment efficacy, enabling timely adjustments for better outcomes. Moreover, predicting flares and prognosis using AI models, as suggested by Fliorent (2024), holds promise in enhancing long-term disease management strategies.

According to several studies such as Giansanti (2023) and Jeong et al. (2023), the advancement of AI in dermatology represents a radical shift in healthcare delivery. Dermatologists may probe deeper into disease processes, optimize treatment options, and enhance patient outcomes. The promise of AI in dermatology extends beyond diagnosis and treatment to areas such as telemedicine, as explained by El-Komy et al. (2022), which can overcome gaps in healthcare access and delivery, particularly in distant or underserved locations.

3.2.1 Early Diagnosis and Risk Stratification

3.2.1.1 Automated Image Analysis for Lesion Detection and Classification

The study of skin lesions in psoriasis is increasingly being automated using artificial intelligence systems. They have transformed the industry by providing the accurate and rapid diagnosis of psoriatic lesions. Using AI-powered analysis of patient data, predictive models may be created to anticipate the onset of psoriasis, allowing for preventive interventions and personalized treatment regimens. These technologies have demonstrated amazing accuracy in recognizing and categorizing psoriatic lesions, aiding in early diagnosis, and monitoring disease progression.

Studies by Marosán-Vilimszky et al. [35] and Liu et al. [36] have underlined the relevance of automated image analysis in lesion categorization, with a focus on the function of deep learning (DL) algorithms in improving clinical diagnosis. Clinical diagnoses can be considerably improved by using computational methods such as SkinSwinViT, a lightweight transformer-based solution for multi-class skin lesion classification.

3.2.1.2 AI-Powered Analysis of Patient Data for Predicting Psoriasis Onset

It also focuses on applying artificial intelligence to examine patient data and forecast the beginning of psoriasis [38]. emphasize the crucial necessity of AI in sickness detection, specifically in biomedical engineering, focusing on its potential in early detection systems. Accurate prediction models for automated psoriasis lesion segmentation and body surface area (BSA) assessment may be constructed using machine learning models such as U-net, as proven in the work by [39, 40] utilized AI to analyse patient data and anticipate the progression of psoriasis. The technique even involved image processing, feature extraction, lesion categorization, and parameter extraction.

Healthcare providers can improve their capacity to effectively identify and analyse psoriasis-related skin abnormalities by automating this process with the aid of AI. Furthermore, AI's predictive powers in assessing patient data for psoriasis onset have the potential to revolutionize early identification and intervention tactics, resulting in more successful treatment. Dermatology is set to make substantial advances in psoriasis diagnosis and treatment as powerful AI algorithms and models are developed and implemented.

3.2.2 Personalized Treatment Strategies

3.2.2.1 AI-Driven Phenotyping and Subtyping of Psoriasis

Researchers might divide psoriasis patients into two groups using artificial intelligence phenotyping and subtyping approaches based on a range of characteristics such as genetic, disease, and drug data. Machine learning algorithms were also utilized to study genetic data and predict the chance of developing psoriatic arthritis among psoriasis patients, highlighting the potential of AI in discovering various categories within the psoriasis spectrum.

Furthermore, the application of artificial intelligence in phenotyping and subtyping psoriasis has proved significant implications for tailored treatment process. Clinicians can better predict illness development and tailor therapy to individual patients by stratifying them based on unique traits.

3.2.2.2 Machine Learning for Predicting Treatment Response and Tailoring Therapy

Machine learning algorithms can predict individual responses to various therapies by analysing a number of data sources. This predictive capacity enables healthcare practitioners to proactively adjust treatment programmes, ensuring that patients receive the most successful treatment method from the start.

Machine learning algorithms can offer personalized therapy methods that maximize efficacy while minimizing adverse effects, taking into consideration unique patient features such as genetic predispositions and illness severity. This individualized treatment plan indicates a change in psoriasis therapy towards precision medicine, which takes into account each patient's specific demands.

3.2.2.3 AI-Assisted Decision Support Systems for Clinicians

These systems employ machine learning algorithms to assess essential patient data, such as genetic profiles, treatment histories, and clinical findings, and then deliver evidence-based recommendations. AI technology helps physicians provide more personalized and effective medicine by synthesizing complicated data and spotting patterns that humans may ignore.

Furthermore, AI-assisted decision support systems have the potential to improve clinical workflows and resource allocation in psoriasis treatment. By automating functions including treatment planning, monitoring, and follow-up, these systems can improve overall patient outcomes. Furthermore, by combining real-time data and patient input, AI systems enable continual learning and modification, ensuring that treatment techniques are current and in line with the most recent evidence-based procedures.

3.2.3 Psoriasis Monitoring and Prognosis

3.2.3.1 Utilizing Wearable Devices and AI for Disease Activity Tracking

Psoriasis makes it challenging to track disease development and anticipate outcomes. Recent technological breakthroughs, notably artificial intelligence (AI), hold immense potential for improving psoriasis treatment. Wearable sensors are one significant use of AI in psoriasis care. They measure disease activity. These sensors, when paired with AI algorithms, can give real-time data on skin temperature, moisture levels, and physical activity, therefore enhancing our understanding of disease progression.

3.2.3.2 AI-Based Analysis of Imaging Data to Monitor Treatment Efficacy

Furthermore, AI-driven analysis of imaging data gives a novel way to assess therapy success in psoriasis patients. Healthcare professionals can better identify changes in skin lesions by using machine learning algorithms to examine imaging modalities such as dermoscopy or ultrasound. This technique not only enhances treatment evaluation precision but also allows for early detection of treatment response or potential side effects.

3.2.3.3 Predicting Flares and Prognosis Using AI Models

Furthermore, AI models can forecast flares and the prognosis in psoriasis patients. AI algorithms can forecast sickness exacerbations by analysing vast volumes of patient data based on various factors. This enables healthcare practitioners to fine-tune treatment plans and enhance patient outcomes. In terms of psoriasis therapy, the use of AI marks a substantial shift in how healthcare practitioners approach the ailment. This transition from a broad strategy to a tailored treatment plan has the potential to enhance psoriasis treatment, providing patients with better outcomes and a greater quality of life.

3.3 Practical Considerations and Future Directions

3.3.1 Integrating AI into Clinical Workflow

Integration of artificial intelligence has been proven to be of utmost significance in the modern-day medicine with many studies highlighting the benefits of AI in enhancing efficiency, precision, and overall patient care. Psoriasis is one of the most frequently occurring dermatological ailments with a global prevalence of 2–3% and a significant economic burden associated with treatment and management of the disease. AI models, specifically machine learning (ML) applications, can be used to improvise the precise evaluation of the skin images, predict complications, and help optimize therapeutic choices most appropriately. This section will delve into areas where AI can be incorporated into clinical workflow.

3.3.1.1 Enhanced Diagnosis and Classification

AI and ML can be used in particular to improve the existing ways to diagnose as well as classify the disease. AI can analyse the skin images of the patients and can differentiate it from other skin disorders. Convolutional neural networks (CNNs) in particular can be used to improve the differential diagnosis with studies indicating better diagnostic results. Similar AI and ML tools have also been used to predict the severity of the disease, thereby aiding and expediting the diagnosis and clinical decision-making process.

3.3.1.2 Personalized Treatment Plan

Biomarkers such as ADAM23, GJB2, and IRS1 involved in the disease progression have been identified with the aid of various machine learning models in conjunction with the RNA sequencing. The AI can help make rationale clinical decision by analysing patient's past medical history and genetic information and can also aid in identification of drug-drug interactions and predict long-term responses and new therapies. Machine learning model has also been used to predict the efficacy of phototherapy in management of psoriasis with sensitivity as high as 84%.

3.3.1.3 Patient Education and Long-Term Management

AI tools and software can be utilized for teleconsultation as well as improving adherence to therapy and remote management of patients undergoing treatment. Utilization of AI chatbot can be done specifically in geriatric patient to improve their adherence to therapy as well as resolve any queries pertaining to the disease therapies.

3.3.2 Data Privacy and Security in AI Applications for Psoriasis

In the healthcare domain, data privacy and security are of paramount importance especially when integrating AI into clinical workflows. The patient identity and confidentiality should be maintained efficiently to prevent data breaches and misuse.

3.3.2.1 Current Landscape of Data Privacy in AI for Psoriasis

Use of artificial intelligence and machine learning in dermatology is largely dependent on the datasets of patient information comprising mainly clinical images, genetic information, and treatment responses. The use of AI and ML is promising specially in improving the entire treatment process for patients suffering from psoriasis, but data safety and privacy act as the biggest barriers to successful implementation of this application into routine practice.

3.3.2.1.1 Regulatory Frameworks and Compliance

To prioritize and safeguard patients, AI applications must adhere and comply with various regulations laid down by regulatory bodies such as General Data Protection Regulation (GDPR), the Health Insurance Portability and Accountability Act (HIPAA), etc. which mandate strict control over the collection, storage, and sharing of health records and utilization of the patient health records. Compliance must also involve implementation of measures such as data anonymization wherein patients are identified based on computer-allocated numbers or sequences rather than names, encryption, and strict access controls.

3.3.2.1.2 Data Anonymization and Encryption

Anonymization process involves stripping data of personally identifiable information (PII) to ensure that individuals cannot be identified. This process is crucial in generating datasets that can be used for AI training without compromising patient privacy. Data anonymization is synonymous with data masking wherein various techniques like tokenization, format-preserving encryption, etc. are used and helps to retain the data for AI research and development while safeguarding patient privacy. Encryption is the process whereby the data generated and stored by AI, its transmission, and its use are not accessed by unauthorized personnel or party. Both anonymization and encryption requirements for successful AI research implementation (*Data Masking and Data Anonymization for Healthcare AI and ML | iTech*, no date).

3.3.3 Explainability and Trust in AI-Based Psoriasis Management

AI-based systems play an important role in improving psoriasis management by providing objective severity assessments and decision support. However, for widespread adoption, it is crucial to address issues of explainability and trust. Explainable AI (XAI) method can help make AI models more transparent and interpretable. AI models can make predictions from the available resources with appropriate explanation to the rationale behind choosing a treatment over others which can indeed increase the trust and acceptance of this application into routine clinical practice.

Study conducted by Huang et al. [34] showed that AI was able to draw Psoriasis Area and Severity Index (PASI) which was subjectively done by dermatologists previously. The AI model demonstrated success in predicting PASI scores, outperforming dermatologists by 33.42%. Its estimates had a significantly lower mean average error, with predicted values closely aligning with those of expert dermatologists.

3.3.4 Emerging Trends in AI for Psoriasis Research

3.3.4.1 Objective Patient Assessment

AI models have already been used in assessing various skin conditions including psoriasis, and various applications are already developed that can perform objective skin image analysis and effectively predict the severity of the disease. Research has also seen immense advancement with respect to the use of therapy design with this data from the image analysis as now the clinical decision-making can be expedited from such model being incorporated.

3.3.4.2 Diagnosis and Evaluation

Diagnosis of psoriasis is made much easier with the use of AI using clinical and dermoscopic images. The use of deep learning model is being developed currently to not merely give the severity assessment of the disease but rather provide a more focused diagnostic assistance.

3.3.4.3 Natural Language Program (NLP)

Recent studies have evaluated the performance of ChatGPT4, a commercial NLP AI platform that analysed unstructured electronic medical records data of psoriasis patients. NLP can help extract insights from large volumes of text data to support research and clinical decision-making.

AI in psoriasis management enhances diagnostics, personalizes treatments, and improves monitoring. CNNs and ML models optimize therapeutic choices. Explainable AI builds trust and supports clinical adoption. Emerging trends in patient assessment, diagnostics, and NLP promise a bright future for AI in dermatological care (Table 3.1).

Table 3.1 Traditional vs. AI-enhanced psoriasis management

Aspect	Traditional psoriasis management	AI-enhanced psoriasis management
Diagnosis	Manual examination and biopsy	Automated image analysis and prediction
Treatment planning	Standardized treatment protocols	Personalized treatment plans based on AI analysis
Patient monitoring	Periodic in-person visits	Continuous monitoring via mobile apps and wearables
Data handling	Manual data entry and storage	Automated data collection and secure cloud storage
Predictive analytics	Limited predictive capabilities	Advanced predictive models for disease progression
Explainability	Clinician explains based on experience	AI provides visual and data-driven explanations
Trust and adoption	High trust in clinician's judgment	Building trust through transparent AI models
Privacy and security	Basic security measures	Advanced encryption and anonymization

3.4 AI Techniques and Technologies in Dermatology

Psoriasis is an autoimmune disorder that causes chronic skin inflammation, which in turn causes discomfort, disfigurement, and functional impairment. Red, scale-covered spots on the skin are a telltale sign of the illness. Roughly 125 million people across the globe deal with a skin problem wherein the patches can aggravate at times. Skin disorders are a major concern for people all over the world, and dermatologists sometimes find it challenging to diagnose these conditions. It is possible that current approaches for detecting these diseases are too complicated, costly, or otherwise unattainable in environments with limited resources. Misdiagnoses put a burden on healthcare systems and can have serious effects on patient health. To maximize diagnostic efficiency and accuracy, a better, more accessible method is required.

Electronic health records (EHRs) and other medical technology are becoming increasingly commonplace, which has led to a significant rise in the amount of data generated by the medical industry. A branch of AI known as machine learning (ML) uses data pattern recognition to teach computers new skills, and this massive dataset is ideal for this purpose. When it comes to machine learning (ML), the visually intensive subject of dermatology is at the forefront, especially in the area of automated medical picture interpretation.

Dermatologists have been able to use a number of machine learning algorithms to successfully diagnose and classify several skin conditions (Table 3.2).

Medical image analysis, and more especially psoriasis diagnosis, stands to benefit greatly from the most recent advancements in deep learning algorithms. When it comes to the problem of differentiating psoriasis from normal skin or other skin conditions, deep learning models provide significant advantages over conventional approaches. A lot of work has gone into determining how severe psoriasis is, but recently there has been an effort to develop automatic detection systems that can beat the results of human specialists' manual assessments. Multiple research studies

Table 3.2 A few models that have been developed for the goal of skin lesion identification by image classification targeting the skin

Model	Strength	Weakness
Support vector machine (SVM) model [72]	Great accuracy and feature handling capabilities	Slow and requires a lot of processing time
Convolutional neural network (CNN) [73]	This system is characterized by its high level of precision and its specific focus on processing image data	It requires a lot of computer power and extensive training data
Long short-term memory (LSTM) model [74]	Improved diagnosis and individualized treatment are outcomes of this model's remarkable performance in medical image processing, which is due to its ability to remember past information in sequential form (long-term dependencies)	Poor generalizability

have shown that deep learning algorithms can accurately identify psoriasis. Two deep learning algorithms, CNN and LSTM, were the subject of a single study. Eighty per cent of the photos that could be used for categorization were used to train these algorithms. There was an accuracy of 84.2% for the CNN model and a 72.3% for the LSTM model. Another study found that convolutional neural networks (CNNs) for skin disease diagnosis had a test accuracy of 94% in detecting psoriasis.

The way psoriasis is being detected is one example of how the diagnostic criteria for skin disorders are undergoing a major shift right now. While conventional models have made significant strides, our findings discuss the game-changing possibilities of AI and DL in real-world dermatology. These models are not meant to replace the important expertise of dermatologists, despite their reliability and efficiency. On the contrary, they serve as powerful tools for improving decision-making, leading to more accurate diagnoses supported by unique features of skin lesions. The capacity to detect skin diseases earlier in the future will depend on our ability to create powerful algorithms and ensure that these models are seamlessly integrated with electronic health records (EHRs). Improving patient care is just the beginning; this opens up huge possibilities for streamlining healthcare delivery and cutting costs associated with delayed diagnoses.

3.5 AI-Driven Diagnosis and Screening of Psoriasis

Psoriasis is a chronic autoimmune condition that speeds up the growth cycle of skin cells which causes fast-building scaly and thickened single patches with itching and soreness. The condition is an interplay between multiple genetic risk factors and their response to environmental triggers leading to a rogue immune reaction in the skin. The combined effects of increased keratinocyte and endothelial cell proliferation with well-defined inflammation involving antigen-presenting cells (APCs), T cells, monocytes, and macrophages induce characteristic epidermal and vascular hyperplasia in psoriasis lesion. The increased risk for comorbidities, such as cardiovascular disease, which is the primary cause of morbidity and mortality in these patients, further demonstrates the systemic nature of psoriasis. Novel targeted therapy has been made possible by recent improvements in our understanding of the pathophysiology of psoriasis, particularly the involvement of inflammation mediated by interleukin-17. AI-driven screening and diagnosis tools have the potential to completely change how psoriasis is managed because they can help track the disease's course and detect the condition more quickly and accurately.

3.5.1 Automated Image Recognition Systems

Automated image recognition systems have revolutionized the diagnosis and screening of various dermatological conditions, including psoriasis. These systems make use of deep learning techniques and machine learning algorithms to identify psoriatic lesions effectively from skin image data, utilizing the power of artificial intelligence (AI).

Artificial intelligence (AI) algorithms are frequently more accurate in diagnosing skin conditions via scans than conventional practitioners. With this accuracy, the likelihood of a misdiagnosis is decreased and prompt and suitable treatment is guaranteed. They drastically cut down on the amount of time needed for diagnosis by swiftly processing and analysing enormous volumes of photos. AI systems, as opposed to human diagnosticians, offer consistent results, removing variability brought on by weariness, experience, or subjective judgment. In locations with limited access to dermatologists, AI-driven technologies can be used to provide diagnostic services in remote and underserved areas.

Sophisticated dermatological imaging equipment or regular cameras are used to take high-quality pictures of the afflicted skin areas. Medical picture classification of skin illnesses is more difficult due to the intricate development, variable coloration, and data security issues. Preprocessing is done on the photos to improve psoriasis-related characteristics like scaling, redness, and plaque thickness. Psoriatic lesions are the subject of machine learning algorithms that extract pertinent features from the images.

Through surface reflection removal and magnification of the lesions, dermoscopy is an imaging procedure that provides more detailed information than what can be seen with the unaided eye. In the differential diagnosis of psoriasis and papulosquamous skin disorders, it is thought to be a helpful technique. The uniformly spaced dotted vessels over an erythematous background and the white scaling of the lesion are characteristic dermoscopic features of psoriasis.

Convolutional neural networks (CNNs) have been used to classify clinical and dermoscopic pictures in recent years. In order to identify pixel-level representative features, the CNN employs a convolution filter. It then uses the extensive collection of dermoscopic image data and the accompanying diagnosis as input for "end-to-end" training. CNN's strength is its capacity to figure out "what to look for" on its own without human assistance. The CNN's performance was on par with dermatologists when it came to classifying benign and malignant skin cancers using clinical photos and the ResNet-152 model.

A CNN trained on dermoscopic images would perform exceptionally well in identifying psoriasis, which might improve the management of psoriasis in areas with limited medical resources because dermoscopic images provide high-resolution information and psoriasis diagnosis is primarily based on the appearance of the skin lesion. However, the categorization of pigmented skin malignancies is the primary focus of current research for computer-aided detection of skin illnesses. Few academics have studied the detection and severity assessment of psoriasis using clinical photos using artificial intelligence (AI).

3.5.2 AI in Histopathological Analysis

Significant advancements in AI have also been made in histopathology analysis, which is essential for psoriasis diagnosis. In histopathology, skin biopsy samples are examined under a microscope to look for psoriasis-specific characteristics such parakeratosis, inflammatory cell infiltration, and epidermal hyperplasia.

The digitization of whole histological glass slides has led to new developments in tissue-based diagnostics. A virtual slide is a process where microscopic images are shown as an entire digital matrix. The calculation and associated display of visual information that would otherwise be needed for each human observation are made possible by a virtual slide.

AI systems are able to identify minute histopathological alterations that a human eye could overlook, which results in more precise diagnosis. They dramatically cut down on the amount of time needed to analyse and interpret biopsy samples, which speeds up clinical decision-making. They also lessen the possibility of human mistake, yielding outcomes that are more consistent and repeatable. AI systems are able to analyse tissue samples quantitatively, providing accurate assessments of pathological traits that are vital for tracking the course of a disease and the effectiveness of treatment.

Skin biopsy samples are processed and stained to bring attention to the diseased characteristics and pertinent cellular structures. Stained samples are digitally photographed in high quality using sophisticated microscopy methods. The digital photos are modified to improve important characteristics' contrast and visibility. Through the analysis of the pictures, machine learning algorithms are able to recognize and measure problematic characteristics including immune cell infiltration and epidermal thickness. As a result, the AI system offers a thorough diagnostic report that includes a diagnosis based on the data analysis and a quantitative evaluation of abnormal aspects.

3.6 Conclusion

Artificial intelligence has the potential to change psoriatic treatment, bringing about significant advances in diagnosis and management. Additionally, AI-powered technologies (machine learning and deep learning algorithms) are utilized to process medical data such as clinical imaging, genetic data, and patient histories. Screening these potentials can provide possibly enhanced, earlier diagnoses of the particular (i.e. psoriatic) rash route, which is critical in adopting respected early therapeutic systems. Furthermore, AI might anticipate the outcome of different kinds of therapy by assessing patient-specific features, and it may assist in personalized treatment regimens for each individual case, therefore optimizing psoriasis care in general, leading to improved outcomes.

AI does more than only diagnose and personalize treatments. It is also critical in monitoring illness development and adherence to treatment. Wearable devices and mobile health applications powered by artificial intelligence can collect patient data over time, providing real-time insight into disease activity and treatment outcomes. This continuous monitoring aids in real-time adjustments of treatment regimens, ensuring that patients receive the most appropriate care based on their unique requirements at all times. AI may also assist in uncovering novel treatment techniques by mining enormous amounts of data from study findings, identifying medication candidates, and speeding up drug discovery. As a result, not only will AI take the present therapy to new heights, but it can also provide revolutionary treatments that might significantly shift the landscape of psoriasis care.

Remaining Challenges and the Path Forwards

Despite the enormous potential for AI to revolutionize psoriasis therapy, a number of challenges remain. One significant barrier to overcome is the need for large, well-managed datasets that represent a diverse spectrum of patients (rather than simply local populations). Because AI algorithms, like all other programmes, only function on what they have continuously trained on, a lack of variety or bias in the data results in inaccurate predictions and suggestions. To construct AI systems capable of giving equal treatment across all demographics, systematic collection of large and representative datasets is required.

Furthermore, significant validation of AI-generated insights is required prior to their use in clinical practice. This research must give proof of how standardized AI technologies may consistently produce high-quality outcomes that are compliant with clinical recommendations. A problem is also the ethical and regulatory aspects of employing AI in healthcare. This includes worries about data privacy, algorithm transparency, and whether AI may exacerbate existing imbalances in healthcare systems. Clarity in the norms and laws that govern AI usage in healthcare is required to guarantee that technology is utilized responsibly and ethically.

Finally, ongoing investment in and training for healthcare workers is essential to ensure that they are familiar with AI technologies and how they might be used in clinical contexts. This goes from being aware of the risks of AI to accurately interpreting and acting on insights generated by this technology. To advance the area, researchers, physicians, and technologists must collaborate to determine how these technologies might be best applied as healthcare solutions. These parties may work together to solve the challenges and maximize the usefulness of AI in psoriasis care. More research should be directed on building next-generation AI models capable of coping with large and diverse datasets while guaranteeing that their validity is supported by well-defined clinical studies. Efforts should also be undertaken to develop common procedures for data collecting and sharing, which would enable the creation of huge, diverse datasets required for any effective AI. As we solve these challenges, AI will be able to work with psoriasis care professionals, perhaps leading to better patient outcomes and a higher quality of life for the millions of people who suffer from this chronic illness.

References

1. Bakshi H, Nagpal M, Singh M, Dhingra GA, Aggarwal G. Treatment of psoriasis: a comprehensive review of entire therapies. Curr Drug Saf. 2020;15(2):82–104.
2. Mahé E. Childhood psoriasis. Eur J Dermatol EJD. 2016;26(6):537–48.
3. Lee HJ, Kim M. Challenges and future trends in the treatment of psoriasis. Int J Mol Sci. 2023;24(17):13313.
4. Thomas L, Azad J, Takwale A. Management of nail psoriasis. Clin Exp Dermatol. 2021;46(1):3–8.
5. Menter A, Van Voorhees AS, Hsu S. Pustular psoriasis: a narrative review of recent developments in pathophysiology and therapeutic options. Dermatol Ther. 2021;11(6):1917–29.
6. Coates LC, Helliwell PS. Psoriatic arthritis: state of the art review. Clin Med Lond Engl. 2017;17(1):65–70.
7. Bronckers IMGJ, Paller AS, van Geel MJ, van de Kerkhof PCM, Seyger MMB. Psoriasis in children and adolescents: diagnosis, management and comorbidities. Paediatr Drugs. 2015;17(5):373–84.
8. Prinz JC, Choon SE, Griffiths CEM, Merola JF, Morita A, Ashcroft DM, et al. Prevalence, comorbidities and mortality of generalized pustular psoriasis: a literature review. J Eur Acad Dermatol Venereol JEADV. 2023;37(2):256–73.
9. Ibrahim S, Amer A, Nofal H, Abdellatif A. Practical compendium for psoriasis management. Dermatol Ther. 2020;33(2):e13243.
10. Ghafoor R, Patil A, Yamauchi P, Weinberg J, Kircik L, Grabbe S, et al. Treatment of scalp psoriasis. J Drugs Dermatol JDD. 2022;21(8):833–7.
11. Signorovitch JE, Wu EQ, Yu AP, Gerrits CM, Kantor E, Bao Y, et al. Comparative effectiveness without head-to-head trials: a method for matching-adjusted indirect comparisons applied to psoriasis treatment with adalimumab or etanercept. PharmacoEconomics. 2010;28(10):935–45.
12. Huang D, Zhang Y, Kong L, Lu J, Shi Y. Janus kinase inhibitors in autoimmune bullous diseases. Front Immunol. 2023a;14:1220887.
13. Azuaga AB, Ramírez J, Cañete JD. Psoriatic arthritis: pathogenesis and targeted therapies. Int J Mol Sci. 2023;24(5):4901.
14. Merola JF, Qureshi A, Husni ME. Underdiagnosed and undertreated psoriasis: nuances of treating psoriasis affecting the scalp, face, intertriginous areas, genitals, hands, feet, and nails. Dermatol Ther. 2018;31(3):e12589.
15. Ng BCK, Jadon DR. Unmet needs in psoriatic arthritis. Best Pract Res Clin Rheumatol. 2021;35(2):101693.
16. Pinson R, Sotoodian B, Fiorillo L. Psoriasis in children. Psoriasis Auckl NZ. 2016;6:121–9.
17. Canal-García E, Bosch-Amate X, Belinchón I, Puig L. Nail Psoriasis. Actas Dermosifiliogr. 2022;113(5):481–90.
18. Ji C, Wang H, Bao C, Zhang L, Ruan S, Zhang J, et al. Challenge of nail psoriasis: an update review. Clin Rev Allergy Immunol. 2021;61(3):377–402.
19. Hwang JK, Grover C, Iorizzo M, Lebwohl MG, Piraccini BM, Rigopoulos DG, et al. Nail psoriasis and nail lichen planus: updates on diagnosis and management. J Am Acad Dermatol. 2024;90(3):585–96.
20. Gottlieb AB, Merola JF. Axial psoriatic arthritis: an update for dermatologists. J Am Acad Dermatol. 2021;84(1):92–101.
21. Napolitano M, Caso F, Scarpa R, Megna M, Patrì A, Balato N, et al. Psoriatic arthritis and psoriasis: differential diagnosis. Clin Rheumatol. 2016;35(8):1893–901.
22. Haberman RH, MacFarlane KA, Catron S, Samuels J, Blank RB, Toprover M, et al. Efficacy of guselkumab, a selective IL-23 inhibitor, in Preventing Arthritis in a Multicentre Psoriasis At-Risk cohort (PAMPA): protocol of a randomised, double-blind, placebo controlled multicentre trial. BMJ Open. 2022;12(12):e063650.
23. Chen L, Tsai TF. HLA-Cw6 and psoriasis. Br J Dermatol. 2018;178(4):854–62.

24. Ford AR, Siegel M, Bagel J, Cordoro KM, Garg A, Gottlieb A, et al. Dietary recommendations for adults with psoriasis or psoriatic arthritis from the medical board of the national psoriasis foundation: a systematic review. JAMA Dermatol. 2018;154(8):934–50.
25. Carrascosa JM, Bonanad C, Dauden E, Botella R, Olveira-Martín A, en nombre del Grupo de Trabajo en Inflamación Sistémica en Psoriasis. Psoriasis and nonalcoholic fatty liver disease. Actas Dermosifiliogr. 2017;108(6):506–14.
26. Sinclair R, Thirthar PV. Tildrakizumab for the treatment of psoriasis. Expert Rev Clin Immunol. 2019;15(1):5–12.
27. Serrano L, Maloney V, Gordon KB. Risankizumab in moderate-to-severe plaque psoriasis. Immunotherapy. 2019;11(16):1357–70.
28. Benoit S, Hamm H. Childhood psoriasis. Clin Dermatol. 2007;25(6):555–62.
29. Tollefson MM. Diagnosis and management of psoriasis in children. Pediatr Clin N Am. 2014;61(2):261–77.
30. Jugovac V, Gulin M, Barić D, Ledić Drvar D, Čeović R. Treatment of plaque-psoriasis in HIV-positive patients. Acta Dermatovenerol Alp Pannonica Adriat. 2024;33(1):37–40.
31. Fujita H, Gooderham M, Romiti R. Diagnosis of generalized pustular psoriasis. Am J Clin Dermatol. 2022;23(Suppl 1):31–8.
32. Zhu CY, Wang YK, Chen HP, Gao KL, Shu C, Wang JC, et al. A deep learning based framework for diagnosing multiple skin diseases in a clinical environment. Front Med. 2021;8:626369.
33. Yu K, Syed MN, Bernardis E, Gelfand JM. Machine learning applications in the evaluation and management of psoriasis: a systematic review. J Psoriasis Psoriatic Arthritis. 2020;5(4):147–59.
34. Huang K, Wu X, Li Y, Lv C, Yan Y, Wu Z, et al. Artificial intelligence–based psoriasis severity assessment: real-world study and application. J Med Internet Res. 2023b;25:e44932.
35. Marosán-Vilimszky P, Szalai K, Horváth A, Csabai D, Füzesi K, Csány G, et al. Automated skin lesion classification on ultrasound images. Diagnostics. 2021;11(7):1207.
36. Liu Z, Wang X, Ma Y, Lin Y, Wang G. Artificial intelligence in psoriasis: where we are and where we are going. Exp Dermatol. 2023;32(11):1884–99.
37. Tang K, Su J, Chen R, Huang R, Dai M, Li Y. SkinSwinViT: a lightweight transformer-based method for multiclass skin lesion classification with enhanced generalization capabilities. Appl Sci. 2024;14(10):4005.
38. Mahmoud NM, Soliman AM. Early automated detection system for skin cancer diagnosis using artificial intelligent techniques. Sci Rep. 2024;14(1):9749.
39. Lin YL, Huang A, Yang CY, Chang WY. Measurement of body surface area for psoriasis using U-net models. Tsui PH, editor. Comput Math Methods Med. 2022;2022:1–9.
40. Martínez-Torres J, Silva Piñeiro A, Alesanco Á, Pérez-Rey I, García J. Automatic image characterization of psoriasis lesions. Mathematics. 2021;9(22):2974.
41. Patrick MT, Stuart PE, Raja K, Gudjonsson JE, Tejasvi T, Yang J, et al. Genetic signature to provide robust risk assessment of psoriatic arthritis development in psoriasis patients. Nat Commun. 2018;9(1):4178.
42. Du AX, Emam S, Gniadecki R. Review of machine learning in predicting dermatological outcomes. Front Med. 2020;7:266.
43. Yao P, Jia Y, Kan X, Chen J, Xu J, Xu H, et al. Identification of ADAM23 as a potential signature for psoriasis using integrative machine-learning and experimental verification. Int J Gen Med. 2023;16:6051–64.
44. Patrick MT, Raja K, Miller K, Sotzen J, Gudjonsson JE, Elder JT, et al. Drug repurposing prediction for immune-mediated cutaneous diseases using a word-embedding–based machine learning approach. J Invest Dermatol. 2019;139(3):683–91.
45. Hong J, Mosca M, Hadeler E, Hakimi M, Bhutani T, Liao W. The future of personalized medicine in psoriasis. Dermatol Rev. 2021;2(5):282–8.
46. Elmets CA, Korman NJ, Prater EF, Wong EB, Rupani RN, Kivelevitch D, et al. Joint AAD–NPF guidelines of care for the management and treatment of psoriasis with topical therapy and alternative medicine modalities for psoriasis severity measures. J Am Acad Dermatol. 2021;84(2):432–70.

47. Jutzi TB, Krieghoff-Henning EI, Holland-Letz T, Utikal JS, Hauschild A, Schadendorf D, et al. Artificial intelligence in skin cancer diagnostics: the patients' perspective. Front Med [Internet]. 2020 Jun 2 [cited 2024 Jun 30];7. Available from: https://www.frontiersin.org/journals/medicine/articles/10.3389/fmed.2020.00233/full.
48. Damiani G, Bragazzi NL, Karimkhani Aksut C, Wu D, Alicandro G, McGonagle D, et al. The global, regional, and national burden of psoriasis: results and insights from the Global Burden of Disease 2019 Study. Front Med. 2021;8:743180.
49. Roslan R, INM R, Sabri N, Ibrahim Z. Evaluation of psoriasis skin disease classification using convolutional neural network. IAES Int J Artif Intell IJ-AI. 2020;9(2):349–55.
50. Yang Y, Wang J, Xie F, Liu J, Shu C, Wang Y, et al. A convolutional neural network trained with dermoscopic images of psoriasis performed on par with 230 dermatologists. Comput Biol Med. 2021;139:104924.
51. Okamoto T, Kawai M, Ogawa Y, Shimada S, Kawamura T. Artificial intelligence for the automated single-shot assessment of psoriasis severity. J Eur Acad Dermatol Venereol. 2022;36(12):2512–5.
52. Xing L, Wu T, Yu L, Zhou N, Zhang Z, Pu Y, et al. Exploration of biomarkers of psoriasis through combined multiomics analysis. Mediat Inflamm. 2022;2022(1):7731082.
53. Tomalin LE, Kim J, Correa da Rosa J, Lee J, Fitz LJ, Berstein G, et al. Early quantification of systemic inflammatory proteins predicts long-term treatment response to tofacitinib and etanercept. J Invest Dermatol. 2020;140(5):1026–34.
54. Narbutt J, Krzyścin J, Sobolewski P, Skibińska M, Noweta M, Owczarek W, et al. A priori estimation of the narrow-band UVB phototherapy outcome for moderate-to-severe psoriasis based on the patients' questionnaire and blood tests using random forest classifier. Clin Cosmet Investig Dermatol. 2021;14:253–9.
55. Sigurgeirsson B, Browning J, Tyring S, Szepietowski JC, Rivera-Díaz R, Effendy I, et al. Secukinumab demonstrates efficacy, safety, and tolerability upon administration by 2 ml autoinjector in adult patients with plaque psoriasis: 52-week results from MATURE, a randomized, placebo-controlled trial. Dermatol Ther. 2022;35(3):e15285.
56. Lunge SB, Shetty NS, Sardesai VR, Karagaiah P, Yamauchi PS, Weinberg JM, et al. Therapeutic application of machine learning in psoriasis: a PRISMA systematic review. J Cosmet Dermatol. 2023;22(2):378–82.
57. Havelin A, Hampton P. Telemedicine and e-Health in the management of psoriasis: improving patient outcomes—a narrative review. Psoriasis Targets Ther. 2022;12:15–24.
58. Omiye JA, Gui H, Daneshjou R, Cai ZR, Muralidharan V. Principles, applications, and future of artificial intelligence in dermatology. Front Med. 2023;10:1278232.
59. McKee M, Wouters OJ. The challenges of regulating artificial intelligence in healthcare. Int J Health Policy Manag. 2022;12:7261.
60. Palaniappan K, Lin EYT, Vogel S. Global regulatory frameworks for the use of Artificial Intelligence (AI) in the healthcare services sector. Healthcare. 2024;12(5):562.
61. Almalawi A, Khan AI, Alsolami F, Abushark YB, Alfakeeh AS. Managing security of healthcare data for a modern healthcare system. Sensors. 2023;23(7):3612.
62. Yadav N, Pandey S, Gupta A, Dudani P, Gupta S, Rangarajan K. Data privacy in healthcare: in the era of artificial intelligence. Indian Dermatol Online J. 2023;14(6):788.
63. Hauser K, Kurz A, Haggenmüller S, Maron RC, von Kalle C, Utikal JS, et al. Explainable artificial intelligence in skin cancer recognition: a systematic review. Eur J Cancer. 2022;167:54–69.
64. Mayanja J, Asanda EH, Mwesigwa J, Tumwebaze P, Marvin G. Explainable artificial intelligence and deep transfer learning for skin disease diagnosis. In: Shakya S, Tavares JMRS, Fernández-Caballero A, Papakostas G, editors. Fourth International Conference on Image Processing and Capsule Networks. Singapore: Springer Nature; 2023a. p. 711–24.
65. Nikam RV, Gowtham M, More PS, Shinde AS. Current and emerging prospects in the psoriatic treatment. Int Immunopharmacol. 2023;120:110331.
66. Shapiro J, Baum S, Pavlotzky F, Mordechai YB, Barzilai A, Freud T, et al. Application of an NLP AI tool in psoriasis: a cross-sectional comparative study on identifying affected areas

in patients' data. Clin Dermatol [Internet]. 2024 Jun 21 [cited 2024 Jun 26]; Available from: https://www.sciencedirect.com/science/article/pii/S0738081X24001020.
67. Armstrong AW, Read C. Pathophysiology, clinical presentation, and treatment of psoriasis: a review. JAMA [Internet]. 2020 May 19 [cited 2024 Jun 23];323(19):1945. Available from: https://jamanetwork.com/journals/jama/fullarticle/2766169.
68. Mayanja J, Asanda EH, Mwesigwa J, Tumwebaze P, Marvin G. Explainable artificial intelligence and deep transfer learning for skin disease diagnosis. In: Shakya S, Tavares JMRS, Fernández-Caballero A, Papakostas G, editors. Fourth International Conference on Image Processing and Capsule Networks [Internet], Lecture Notes in Networks and Systems; vol. 798. Singapore: Springer Nature Singapore; 2023b [cited 2024 Jun 23]. p. 711–724. Available from: https://link.springer.com/10.1007/978-981-99-7093-3_47.
69. Fujisawa Y, Otomo Y, Ogata Y, Nakamura Y, Fujita R, Ishitsuka Y, et al. Deep-learning-based, computer-aided classifier developed with a small dataset of clinical images surpasses board-certified dermatologists in skin tumour diagnosis. Br J Dermatol [Internet]. 2019 Feb [cited 2024 Jun 23];180(2):373–81. Available from: https://academic.oup.com/bjd/article/180/2/373/6601593.
70. Haenssle HA, Fink C, Schneiderbauer R, Toberer F, Buhl T, Blum A, et al. Man against machine: diagnostic performance of a deep learning convolutional neural network for dermoscopic melanoma recognition in comparison to 58 dermatologists. Ann Oncol [Internet]. 2018 Aug [cited 2024 Jun 23];29(8):1836–1842. Available from: https://linkinghub.elsevier.com/retrieve/pii/S0923753419341055.
71. Han SS, Kim MS, Lim W, Park GH, Park I, Chang SE. Classification of the clinical images for benign and malignant cutaneous tumors using a deep learning algorithm. J Invest Dermatol [Internet]. 2018 Jul [cited 2024 Jun 23];138(7):1529–1538. Available from: https://linkinghub.elsevier.com/retrieve/pii/S0022202X18301118.
72. Pereira S, Joshi U. Implementation of support vector machine technique in feedback analysis system. Int J Comput Appl [Internet]. 2014 Jun 18 [cited 2024 Jun 23];96(17):24–8. Available from: http://research.ijcaonline.org/volume96/number17/pxc3896906.pdf.
73. Thiele F, Windebank AJ, Siddiqui AM. Motivation for using data-driven algorithms in research: a review of machine learning solutions for image analysis of micrographs in neuroscience. J Neuropathol Exp Neurol [Internet]. 2023 Jun 20 [cited 2024 Jun 24];82(7):595–610. Available from: https://journals.lww.com/10.1093/jnen/nlad040.
74. Li M, Jiang Y, Zhang Y, Zhu H. Medical image analysis using deep learning algorithms. Front Public Health [Internet]. 2023 Nov 7 [cited 2024 Jun 25];11:1273253. Available from: https://www.frontiersin.org/articles/10.3389/fpubh.2023.1273253/full.
75. Aijaz SF, Khan SJ, Azim F, Shakeel CS, Hassan U. Deep learning application for effective classification of different types of psoriasis. Hasikin K, editor. J Healthc Eng [Internet]. 2022a Jan 15 [cited 2024 Jun 25];2022:1–12. Available from: https://www.hindawi.com/journals/jhe/2022/7541583/.
76. Amin N, Farooq MS. Automated psoriasis detection using deep learning. VFAST Trans Softw Eng [Internet]. 2021 Sep 30 [cited 2024 Jun 25];9(3):93–101. Available from: https://vfast.org/journals/index.php/VTSE/article/view/686.
77. Aijaz SF, Khan SJ, Azim F, Shakeel CS, Hassan U. Deep learning application for effective classification of different types of psoriasis. Hasikin K, editor. J Healthc Eng. 2022b;2022:1–12.
78. Hawkes JE, Chan TC, Krueger JG. Psoriasis pathogenesis and the development of novel targeted immune therapies. J Allergy Clin Immunol. 2017;140(3):645–53.
79. McCormick T, Ayala-Fontanez N, Soler D. Current knowledge on psoriasis and autoimmune diseases. Psoriasis Targets Ther. 2016;7
80. Hossen MN, Panneerselvam V, Koundal D, Ahmed K, Bui FM, Ibrahim SM. Federated machine learning for detection of skin diseases and enhancement of Internet of Medical Things (IoMT) security. IEEE J Biomed Health Inform. 2023;27(2):835–41.
81. Han H, Li Y, Zhu X. Convolutional neural network learning for generic data classification. Inf Sci. 2019;477:448–65.

82. Kayser K, GĂśrtler J, Bogovac M, Bogovac A, Goldmann T, Vollmer E, et al. AI (artificial intelligence) in histopathology--from image analysis to automated diagnosis. Folia Histochem Cytobiol. 2010;47(3):355–61.
83. Štifanic J, Štifanić D, Zulijani A, Car Z. Application of AI in histopathological image analysis. In: Filipovic N, editor. Applied artificial intelligence: medicine, biology, chemistry, financial, games, engineering [Internet], Lecture Notes in Networks and Systems, vol. 659. Cham: Springer International Publishing; 2023. p. 121–31. Available from: https://link.springer.com/10.1007/978-3-031-29717-5_9.
84. Esteva A, Kuprel B, Novoa RA, Ko J, Swetter SM, Blau HM, et al. Dermatologist-level classification of skin cancer with deep neural networks. Nature. 2017;542(7639):115–8.
85. Tschandl P, Rinner C, Apalla Z, Argenziano G, Codella N, Halpern A, et al. Human–computer collaboration for skin cancer recognition. Nat Med. 2020;26(8):1229–34.
86. Brinker TJ, Hekler A, Enk AH, Klode J, Hauschild A, Berking C, et al. Deep learning outperformed 136 of 157 dermatologists in a head-to-head dermoscopic melanoma image classification task. Eur J Cancer. 2019;113:47–54.

4 The Role of Artificial Intelligence in Skin Cancer Detection: Advancements and Challenges

Qasi Najah, Nereen A. Almosilhy, and Esraa M. AlEdani

4.1 Overview of Nonmelanoma Skin Cancers: BCC and SCC

Skin cancer is broadly divided into two groups: nonmelanoma skin cancers and melanoma. Nonmelanoma skin cancers are further subdivided into basal cell carcinoma (BCC) and squamous cell carcinoma (SCC). BCC is the most common type of skin cancer for approximately 80% of cases. It develops from basal cells in the deepest layer of the epidermis. If left untreated, BCC can cause extensive damage to the affected skin. Although BCC tends to grow slowly and rarely metastasizes, it can still cause significant local damage, especially in delicate areas such as the face and arms. BCC typically presents as a pearly translucent nodule, but it can also appear as a white, wax-like scar or a flat, scaly lesion. While less aggressive than melanoma, BCC still requires proper diagnosis and treatment. On the other hand, SCC accounts for about 20% of all skin cancers and originates from squamous cells, which make up most of the skin's upper layers. SCC commonly occurs on sun-exposed areas of the body, such as the face, ears, neck, lips, and backs of the hands. It can manifest as a scaly patch, a raised bump with scabbing or crusting, or an ulcer that may bleed. Early detection and treatment are essential, as SCC has a higher potential for metastasis to distant sites compared to BCC. While SCC is less common than melanoma, it can become a life-threatening condition if left to progress.

Q. Najah
Elmergib University, Alkhums, Libya

N. A. Almosilhy (✉)
Department of Pharmacology and Toxicology, Faculty of Pharmacy, Tanta University, Tanta, Egypt

E. M. AlEdani
University of Basrah, College of Medicine, Basra, Iraq

E. M. AlEdani, H. I. Maibach (eds.), *Applications of Artificial Intelligence in Common Dermatological Diseases*, Updates in Clinical Dermatology,
https://doi.org/10.1007/978-3-031-78139-1_4

4.2 Melanoma: The Most Lethal Skin Cancer with Global Impact

Melanoma, a deadly form of skin cancer, accounts for over 80% of skin cancer deaths and originates in melanocytes, the pigment-producing cells in the basal layer of the epidermis. As these melanocytes are derived from the neural crest, they can produce signaling molecules that encourage migration and metastasis following malignant transformation. Melanoma often appears as a patch with notched, blurred, or irregular edges. Although it represents only 1% of skin cancer cases, it is the most lethal, causing around 55,500 deaths worldwide each year. However, incidence and mortality rates vary globally, with the highest reported in New Zealand and Australia.

4.3 Key Risk Factors for Skin Cancer

Risk factors associated with skin cancer include exposure to UV radiation, possessing fair skin tone, and a family history of skin cancer. Other risk factors include having multiple or atypical moles, a history of sunburns, or a weakened immune system. Additionally, hereditary diseases like xeroderma pigmentosum, which impair the skin cells' ability to repair UV damage, significantly increase the risk of developing skin cancer.

4.4 Genomics and New Treatments for Skin Cancer

Advances in genomics have significantly improved our understanding of the molecular and signaling pathways underlying skin cancer etiology. For instance, a mutation in the hedgehog signaling pathway has been identified as a contributing cause of basal cell carcinoma. This finding has led to the development of new pathway inhibitors, now used in treating advanced or metastatic BCCs that are nonresponsive to radiation or surgery. Similarly, mutations in the BRAF gene associated with malignant melanoma have resulted in the discovery of targeted therapies that selectively inhibit the activity of the mutated BRAF protein.

4.5 Skin Cancer Detection: Comparing Visual Inspection and Dermoscopy

Diagnosis of skin cancer begins with a visual examination by a dermatologist. However, this technique is subjective and primarily relies on the clinician's experience and expertise in evaluating suspicious patterns and signs of skin cancer, such as asymmetry, border irregularity, color variation, diameter, and evolution—collectively known as the ABCDE criteria. A conclusive diagnosis cannot be made based only on visual inspection with the naked eye; histopathological examination is necessary in all instances. In cases where access to a specialized dermatologist is unavailable, relying only on a physician's examination in primary care could lead to missed early melanomas and atypical presentations, which carry the risk of false negatives, leading to missed diagnoses, as well as false positives, potentially resulting in unnecessary biopsies.

Dermoscopy is a practical, noninvasive technique that uses a light source and a magnifying lens to visualize skin lesions in detail, aiding in the early detection of skin cancers. It makes subclinical structures of the skin more detectable, allowing for the identification of subtle features indicative of skin cancer. Digital dermoscopy devices, on the other hand, capture images of skin lesions and apply computer algorithms to these images, thereby improving diagnostic capabilities for skin cancer detection. Additionally, digital dermoscopy can automatically assist in diagnosis using artificial intelligence (AI) and save images for monitoring over time. Compared to visual inspection with the naked eye, dermoscopy enhances diagnostic accuracy and allows for more precise documentation, as digital tools can record and compare images over time. However, dermoscopy and digital dermoscopy systems do have some drawbacks. For example, dermoscopy has a steep learning curve and requires extensive training, while digital systems involve significant economic costs and require specialized equipment and software.

4.6 The Evolution and Impact of AI in Skin Cancer Diagnosis

In the era of artificial intelligence, leveraging the advanced capabilities of AI could be a game-changer in the diagnosis of skin cancers, as it can be easy to use, cost-effective, and increasingly accessible in resource-limited economies. The use of AI in diagnosing skin cancer dates to the early 2000s. In 2002, researchers examined the potential of digital dermoscopy and artificial neural networks for improving the diagnosis of atypically pigmented skin lesions. They used a computerized analysis of digital images, which led to a 93% accuracy rate in differentiating melanoma from benign lesions. However, at that time, restrictions in computing power made the widespread use of neural networks impractical.

Significant advancements in AI development were facilitated by the release of Compute Unified Device Architecture (CUDA), a parallel computing platform and programming model created by NVIDIA in 2007. CUDA allows developers to use NVIDIA's graphics processing units (GPUs), which are specialized electronic circuits designed to accelerate the processing of images and videos, for general-purpose processing. NVIDIA's CUDA platform empowered researchers to leverage the high-performance capabilities of GPUs for general-purpose programming. This breakthrough enabled significantly faster training of neural networks compared to traditional computer's central processing units (CPUs), making it possible to develop and train complex, deep neural networks such as convolutional neural networks (CNNs).

In 2012, the field of deep learning saw substantial progress with Alex Krizhevsky and colleagues' AlexNet, a deep convolutional neural network that achieved exceptional accuracy in the ImageNet Large Scale Visual Recognition

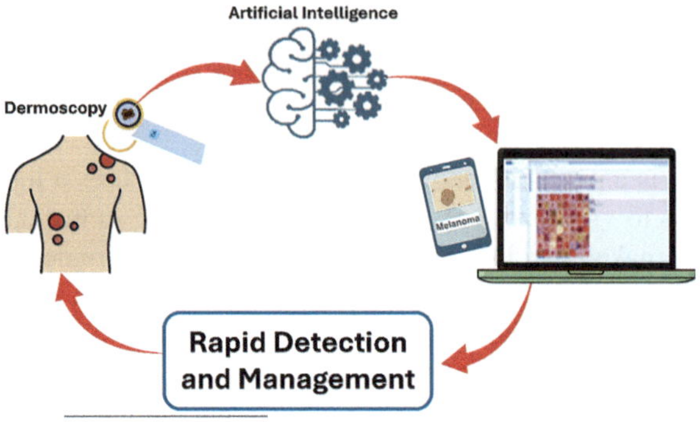

Fig. 4.1 Workflow of artificial intelligence-assisted rapid detection and management of skin lesions using dermoscopy

Challenge. AlexNet's success was attributed to several innovative techniques, including the use of rectified linear units (ReLUs) for faster training, dropout layers to prevent overfitting, and data augmentation to increase the diversity of the training data. These advancements provided a solid foundation for future AI models, enabling them to achieve even greater accuracy and efficiency. Following AlexNet's success, researchers and developers began exploring the application of deep learning in various fields, including dermatology. The ability of AI to analyze complex patterns in large datasets makes it particularly well-suited for medical image analysis. In dermatology, this has led to the development of AI algorithms capable of examining skin lesions and identifying potential malignancies with high precision (Fig. 4.1).

4.7 Clinical Evidence of AI Applications in Skin Cancer Detection

Several studies have explored the application of AI in the detection, diagnosis, and management of skin cancers (Table 4.1). Esteva et al. [23] trained a GoogLeNet Inception v3 CNN classifier to classify skin lesions using a dataset of 129,450 clinical images of 2032 diseases. The model achieved a 72.1% accuracy, exceeding the 65.56% and 66.0% accuracies of two dermatologists. They concluded that the deep CNN demonstrated high sensitivity and specificity in diagnosing keratinocyte carcinomas and malignant melanomas, comparable to that of dermatologists, indicating the potential for low-cost, universal access to diagnostic care. Another large study by Brinker et al. [24, 25], published in two articles, employed the residual network CNN (ResNet50 CNN) to classify dermoscopic images of melanomas and atypical nevi (moles). Trained on 12,378 dermoscopic images from the archive of

Table 4.1 Summary of clinical studies integrating artificial intelligence/machine learning in skin cancer detection

Study ID	AI model	Dataset	Key metrics	Conclusion
Esteva et al. [23]	GoogLeNet Inception v3 CNN	129,450 clinical images, consisting of 2032 different diseases	Accuracy: 72%	CNN is capable of classifying skin cancer comparable to dermatologists
Brinker et al. [24, 25]	ResNet50 CNN	12,378 open-source dermoscopic images (ISIC archive)	Specificity: 68.2%	CNN outperformed dermatologists in dermoscopic melanoma classification
Tschandl et al. [26]	139 machine learning (ML) algorithms	10,015 training images, 1511 test images (ISIC 2018 challenge)	Top 3 algorithms: 25.43 correct diagnoses out of 30	ML algorithms outperformed human experts in diagnosing pigmented skin lesions
Maron et al. [27]	Convolutional neural network (CNN)	1200 dermoscopic images (600 melanomas, 600 nevi) from the ISIC archive	Mean sensitivity improvement, 59.4–74.6%; mean accuracy, 65–73.6%	AI assistance improved dermatologists' sensitivity and accuracy in classifying melanomas and nevi
Han et al. [28]	CNN AI model, called Model Dermatology	576 patients with suspicious skin lesions	Diagnostic accuracy: 53.9% (AI-assisted) vs. 43.8% (unaided)	AI assistance improved diagnostic accuracy, especially for non-dermatology trainees, but it did not enhance expert-level accuracy
Menzies et al. [29]	7-class AI, ISIC AI	172 suspicious pigmented lesions (84 malignant) from 124 patients	7-class model: accuracy difference, 1.2% (vs. specialists). ISIC model: accuracy 11.6% lower (vs. specialists)	7-class AI performed equivalently to specialists and was significantly superior to novice clinicians. The ISIC AI, although superior to novices, was inferior to specialists
	7-class-1 AI, 7-class-2 AI, 7-class-3 AI, ISIC-1 AI, ISIC diagnosis management AI	5696 pigmented lesions (18 malignant) from 66 high-risk patients	7-class-3 AI: accuracy difference 0.5% to 0.4% lower (vs. specialists)	7-class management AI was slightly inferior to specialists but outperformed novices in specific scenarios

(continued)

Table 4.1 (continued)

Study ID	AI model	Dataset	Key metrics	Conclusion
Marchetti et al. [30]	ADAE (All Data Are Ext)	603 lesions (95 melanomas) from 435 participants	Sensitivity, 96.8%; specificity, 37.4%	ADAE algorithm showed high sensitivity and moderate specificity for melanoma diagnosis and improved dermatologists' risk assessment
Papachristou et al. [31]	Dermalyser®	253 lesions from 228 patients (21 melanomas)	Sensitivity, 95.2%; specificity, 84.5%; AUROC, 0.960	The AI-based decision support tool showed high diagnostic accuracy when used in primary care settings
Giavina-Bianchi et al. [32]	Dermoscopy model, clinical model	Dermoscopy and clinical images	Dermoscopy model: accuracy, 89.3%; sensitivity, 0.91; specificity, 0.89 Clinical model: accuracy, 84.7%; sensitivity, 0.89; specificity, 0.83. Both models achieved an AUC > 0.9	AI models showed promising performance in primary care melanoma screening

International Skin Imaging Collaboration (ISIC), it was evaluated against 157 dermatologists and achieved a higher specificity of 68.2% compared to the dermatologists' sensitivity of 89.4% and specificity of 64.4%.

Interestingly, Tschandl et al. [26] compared the diagnostic performance of 139 machine learning (ML) algorithms from the ISIC 2018 challenge with that of 511 human readers, including expert dermatologists, dermatology residents, and general practitioners. The ML algorithms, trained on 10,015 images, significantly outperformed the human readers on a test set of 1511 images. The top 3 algorithms achieved 25.43 correct diagnoses out of 30, compared to 18.78 by human readers, and demonstrated higher sensitivity across various lesion types, particularly in detecting malignant conditions like melanoma. These findings support integrating ML algorithms into dermatological practice to enhance diagnostic accuracy and patient outcomes.

Furthermore, Maron et al. [27] studied the influence of an AI support system on dermatologists' classification of melanomas and nevi using 1200 dermoscopic images (600 melanomas, 600 nevi) from the ISIC archive. With CNN AI assistance, dermatologists demonstrated improved sensitivity and accuracy, with mean sensitivity increasing from 59.4% to 74.6% and mean accuracy increasing from 65.0% to 73.6%.

Nevertheless, many of these studies are based on retrospective data, which are susceptible to various biases. Retrospective studies often rely on previously collected data, which might not be representative of the broader patient population, leading to selection bias. Additionally, comparing the performance of AI algorithms with that of dermatologists using only digital images—without clinical history and physical examination—can underestimate the dermatologists' accuracy in detecting malignant skin lesions. Therefore, studies using AI algorithms should be carefully interpreted within the context of these limitations.

In 2020, Han and colleagues conducted the first prospective randomized controlled trial (RCT) in which clinicians used a CNN AI model, Model Dermatology, Build2020, to diagnose skin neoplasms. The study, involving 576 patients at a South Korean tertiary care center, demonstrated that AI assistance significantly improved diagnostic accuracy (53.9% vs. 43.8% in the unaided group), particularly in the non-dermatology trainees' group (54.7% vs. 29.7% in the unaided group). While the AI model enhanced the performance of dermatology trainees to the level of expert dermatologists in retrospective settings, it had a limited impact on dermatology residents in this prospective study. The findings suggest that AI can be a valuable tool for enhancing diagnostic accuracy among non-dermatology specialists in real-world settings.

Another prospective clinical trial by Menzies et al. [29] investigated AI-powered mobile phone applications for diagnosing and managing pigmented skin lesions. The diagnostic trial included 172 suspicious pigmented lesions (84 malignant) from 124 patients, each with 1 or more lesions greater than 3 mm in diameter, who were scheduled for a biopsy. Two AI models were evaluated in this trial: a 7-class AI model and the ISIC AI model. The 7-class model performed similarly to specialists, with only a 1.2% difference in accuracy, and outperformed novice clinicians by 21.5%. In contrast, the ISIC model was less accurate than the specialists, with an 11.6% lower accuracy, but was still more accurate than novice clinicians by 8.7%. The management trial involved 5696 pigmented lesions from 66 high-risk patients. Five AI models were tested, including variations of the 7-class and ISIC AI algorithms. The results showed that the best-performing AI model, the 7-class-3 AI, was slightly inferior to specialists (0.5% to 0.4% difference) but outperformed novice clinicians by 0.4% in specific scenarios.

Additionally, Marchetti et al. [30] assessed the accuracy of the prospective performance of the open-source AI algorithm, ADAE (All Data Are Ext), which was the winner of the ISIC 2020 competition, in diagnosing melanoma and its impact on dermatologists' decision-making using dermoscopy images from 435 participants (603 lesions, 95 melanomas). The AI algorithm demonstrated high sensitivity (96.8%) and moderate specificity (37.4%) at a predetermined threshold. The study also highlighted the improvement in melanoma risk assessment by dermatologists after using the AI algorithm.

Recently, a Swedish prospective clinical trial by Papachristou et al. [31] evaluated the diagnostic performance of Dermalyser®, an AI-based clinical decision support tool operated via a smartphone application for primary care physicians. The algorithm provided a dichotomous decision support text regarding melanoma evidence. The study included 253 lesions of concern in 228 patients, with 21 confirmed melanomas. The app's accuracy was demonstrated by an area under the receiver operating characteristic curve (AUROC) of 0.960, with a sensitivity of 95.2% and a specificity of 84.5%. Notably, for invasive melanomas alone, the AUROC was 0.988, with 100% sensitivity and 92.6% specificity.

Moreover, Bianchi et al. (2021) investigated the potential of using a computer-aided diagnosis system for melanoma screening in a primary care setting. Two AI models were used: one trained on dermoscopy images and the other on clinical images. The dermoscopy model showed an accuracy of 89.3%, a sensitivity of 0.91, and a specificity of 0.89, while the clinical model showed an accuracy of 84.7%, a sensitivity of 0.89, and a specificity of 0.83. Both models reported an AUC above 0.9, reflecting outstanding performance.

4.8 Limitations and Challenges in AI Application for Skin Cancer

Artificial intelligence has shown great promise in enhancing the accuracy of skin cancer diagnosis and treatment in dermatology. However, several challenges remain. Lack of generalizability is one of the significant challenges of applying AI algorithms in skin cancer detection.

4.8.1 Understanding the Challenge of Generalizability in AI Models

Generalizability refers to the ability of an algorithm to maintain acceptable performance across different settings and populations. When a model demonstrates high accuracy on a certain dataset but cannot maintain the same performance in different settings, this limitation is commonly known as overfitting, which can lead to a lack of generalizability. For instance, in the study by Han et al. [28], a retrospective evaluation of their model showed high accuracy in diagnosing skin conditions. However, when the model was applied to prospective data, its performance significantly decreased. The researchers attributed this decrease to the existence of out-of-distribution cases that the model had never been trained on. Another instance of model overfitting is reported by Menzies et al. [29], who found that the ISIC AI model's accuracy dropped significantly when tested on new, prospective, and unseen data.

4.8.2 The Importance of Data Standardization in AI Performance

Furthermore, standardization is a critical concern for the application of AI in the diagnosis of skin cancer, as different lighting conditions, camera quality, and skin tones can significantly impact the diagnostic power of the system. Oloruntoba et al. [34] compared the performance of models trained on standardized versus non-standardized data, derived from a variety of image-capturing devices, and found that the model pre-trained on standardized data significantly outperformed an identical architecture trained on non-standardized data. This finding indicates that data standardization is an essential procedure for optimizing CNN model performance in medical image analysis and diagnostics.

4.8.3 Diverse and Extensive Data Are Crucial for Successful AI Development

In order to develop a reliable AI algorithm, a vast amount of data is likely required for training. Collecting such a large amount of accurately labeled data may pose a significant challenge when using this technology in a clinical setting. To address this challenge, the American Academy of Dermatology (AAD) is currently working to assemble a reliable dataset involving various skin conditions in diverse populations. They initiated the DataDerm project to create a clinical data registry that streamlines data extraction from electronic health records, enhancing care quality with minimal impact on workflows.

4.8.4 The Importance of Metadata in Enhancing AI Diagnostic Accuracy

Similar lesions, such as a new Spitzoid lesion in a child versus one in an elderly individual, can have different clinical significance. However, most imaging databases used for AI training lack metadata, meaning algorithms are trained only on pixel data. Yap et al. [38] demonstrated that adding metadata to images can enhance AI's diagnostic accuracy.

4.8.5 Racial and Ethnic Disparities: Limitations and Challenges in Dermatological AI Research

Racial and ethnic disparities persist as a longstanding issue in dermatological research. The underrepresentation of ethnic minorities and darker skin tones has been reported in several studies. Most studies on AI in skin cancer detection concentrate on fair skin tones, which can introduce biases and inaccuracies for patients with darker skin tones. In a literature review conducted by Fliorent et al. [42] evaluating the current state of AI in skin cancer detection for patients with colored skin, they found that most AI studies in dermatology underrepresented patients with darker skin tones, highlighting the urgent need for more extensive research in this field. To ensure equitable care for all patients, regardless of skin color, efforts to enhance diversity in dermatology need to reach an international level. Global collaboration is vital for driving change and promoting diversity in dermatologic research. Collaboration within the medical community is essential for addressing disparities and ensuring the effectiveness of AI technologies in dermatology for patients of diverse backgrounds.

4.9 Conclusion

In conclusion, artificial intelligence holds tremendous promise in revolutionizing skin cancer detection, diagnosis, and management. AI systems have demonstrated impressive accuracy in identifying skin lesions, sometimes even outperforming experienced dermatologists. This progress opens up the possibility for earlier and more accurate diagnoses, which are crucial for effective treatment and better patient outcomes. Despite the progress, significant challenges and limitations remain. AI models must become more generalizable, performing effectively across various settings and populations. Standardizing the data used to train these models and ensuring diversity in training datasets are critical steps in addressing these issues. Moving forward, ongoing research, collaboration among experts, and comprehensive testing are essential to enhancing AI tools, making them reliable and effective for everyone. With these efforts, AI could become an invaluable asset in the fight against skin cancer, improving diagnostic accuracy and saving lives.

References

1. Miller SJ, Alam M, Andersen J, Berg D, Bichakjian CK, Bowen G, et al. Basal cell and squamous cell skin cancers. J Natl Compr Cancer Netw. 2010;8(8):836–64.
2. Fania L, Didona D, Morese R, Campana I, Coco V, Di Pietro FR, et al. Basal cell carcinoma: from pathophysiology to novel therapeutic approaches. Biomedicines. 2020;8(11):449.
3. Evans D, Ladusans E, Rimmer S, Burnell L, Thakker N, Farndon P. Complications of the naevoid basal cell carcinoma syndrome: results of a population based study. J Med Genet. 1993;30(6):460–4.
4. Elder DE. Skin cancer. Melanoma and other specific nonmelanoma skin cancers. Cancer. 1995;75(S1):245–56.
5. Saginala K, Barsouk A, Aluru JS, Rawla P, Barsouk A. Epidemiology of melanoma. Med Sci. 2021;9(4):63.
6. Arnold M, Singh D, Laversanne M, Vignat J, Vaccarella S, Meheus F, et al. Global burden of cutaneous melanoma in 2020 and projections to 2040. JAMA Dermatol. 2022;158(5):495–503.
7. Gordon R, editor. Skin cancer: an overview of epidemiology and risk factors. Seminars in oncology nursing. Elsevier; 2013.
8. Lehmann AR, McGibbon D, Stefanini M. Xeroderma pigmentosum. Orphanet J Rare Dis. 2011;6:1–6.
9. Bale AE, Yu K-p. The hedgehog pathway and basal cell carcinomas. Hum Mol Genet. 2001;10(7):757–62.
10. Von Hoff DD, LoRusso PM, Rudin CM, Reddy JC, Yauch RL, Tibes R, et al. Inhibition of the hedgehog pathway in advanced basal-cell carcinoma. N Engl J Med. 2009;361(12):1164–72.
11. Ascierto PA, Kirkwood JM, Grob J-J, Simeone E, Grimaldi AM, Maio M, et al. The role of BRAF V600 mutation in melanoma. J Transl Med. 2012;10:1–9.

12. Wellbrock C, Hurlstone A. BRAF as therapeutic target in melanoma. Biochem Pharmacol. 2010;80(5):561–7.
13. Abbasi NR, Shaw HM, Rigel DS, Friedman RJ, McCarthy WH, Osman I, et al. Early diagnosis of cutaneous melanoma: revisiting the ABCD criteria. JAMA. 2004;292(22):2771–6.
14. Ojeda R, Graells J. Effectiveness of primary care physicians and dermatologists in the diagnosis of skin cancer: a comparative study in the same geographic area. Actas Dermosifiliogr (Engl Ed). 2011;102(1):48–52.
15. Campos-do-Carmo G, Ramos-e-Silva M. Dermoscopy: basic concepts. Int J Dermatol. 2008;47(7):712–9.
16. Rajpara S, Botello A, Townend J, Ormerod A. Systematic review of dermoscopy and digital dermoscopy/artificial intelligence for the diagnosis of melanoma. Br J Dermatol. 2009;161(3):591–604.
17. Skvara H, Teban L, Fiebiger M, Binder M, Kittler H. Limitations of dermoscopy in the recognition of melanoma. Arch Dermatol. 2005;141(2):155–60.
18. Rubegni P, Burroni M, Perotti R, Fimiani M, Andreassi L, Cevenini G, et al. Digital dermoscopy analysis and artificial neural network for the differentiation of clinically atypical pigmented skin lesions: a retrospective study. J Invest Dermatol. 2002;119(2):471–4.
19. Shams R, Kennedy R. Efficient histogram algorithms for NVIDIA CUDA compatible devices. In: Proc Int Conf on Signal Processing and Communications Systems (ICSPCS). CiteSeer; 2007.
20. Sanders J, Kandrot E. CUDA by example: an introduction to general-purpose GPU programming. Addison-Wesley Professional; 2010.
21. Alom MZ, Taha TM, Yakopcic C, Westberg S, Sidike P, Nasrin MS, et al. The history began from AlexNet: a comprehensive survey on deep learning approaches. arXiv preprint arXiv:180301164. 2018.
22. Chen H-C, Widodo AM, Wisnujati A, Rahaman M, Lin JC-W, Chen L, et al. AlexNet convolutional neural network for disease detection and classification of tomato leaf. Electronics. 2022;11(6):951.
23. Esteva A, Kuprel B, Novoa RA, Ko J, Swetter SM, Blau HM, et al. Dermatologist-level classification of skin cancer with deep neural networks. Nature. 2017;542(7639):115–8.
24. Brinker TJ, Hekler A, Enk AH, Klode J, Hauschild A, Berking C, et al. A convolutional neural network trained with dermoscopic images performed on par with 145 dermatologists in a clinical melanoma image classification task. Eur J Cancer. 2019a;111:148–54.
25. Brinker TJ, Hekler A, Enk AH, Klode J, Hauschild A, Berking C, et al. Deep learning outperformed 136 of 157 dermatologists in a head-to-head dermoscopic melanoma image classification task. Eur J Cancer. 2019b;113:47–54.
26. Tschandl P, Codella N, Akay BN, Argenziano G, Braun RP, Cabo H, et al. Comparison of the accuracy of human readers versus machine-learning algorithms for pigmented skin lesion classification: an open, web-based, international, diagnostic study. Lancet Oncol. 2019;20(7):938–47.
27. Maron RC, Utikal JS, Hekler A, Hauschild A, Sattler E, Sondermann W, et al. Artificial intelligence and its effect on dermatologists' accuracy in dermoscopic melanoma image classification: web-based survey study. J Med Internet Res. 2020;22(9):e18091.
28. Han SS, Kim YJ, Moon IJ, Jung JM, Lee MY, Lee WJ, et al. Evaluation of artificial intelligence–assisted diagnosis of skin neoplasms: a single-center, paralleled, unmasked, randomized controlled trial. J Invest Dermatol. 2022;142(9):2353–62. e2
29. Menzies SW, Sinz C, Menzies M, Lo SN, Yolland W, Lingohr J, et al. Comparison of humans versus mobile phone-powered artificial intelligence for the diagnosis and management of pigmented skin cancer in secondary care: a multicentre, prospective, diagnostic, clinical trial. Lancet Digit Health. 2023;5(10):e679–e91.
30. Marchetti MA, Cowen EA, Kurtansky NR, Weber J, Dauscher M, DeFazio J, et al. Prospective validation of dermoscopy-based open-source artificial intelligence for melanoma diagnosis (PROVE-AI study). NPJ Digit Med. 2023;6(1):127.

31. Papachristou P, Söderholm M, Pallon J, Taloyan M, Polesie S, Paoli J, et al. Evaluation of an artificial intelligence-based decision support for the detection of cutaneous melanoma in primary care: a prospective real-life clinical trial. Br J Dermatol. 2024;191(1):125–33.
32. Giavina-Bianchi M, de Sousa RM, Paciello VZA, Vitor WG, Okita AL, Prôa R, et al. Implementation of artificial intelligence algorithms for melanoma screening in a primary care setting. PLoS One. 2021;16(9):e0257006.
33. Gomolin A, Netchiporouk E, Gniadecki R, Litvinov IV. Artificial intelligence applications in dermatology: where do we stand? Front Med. 2020;7:100.
34. Oloruntoba AI, Vestergaard T, Nguyen TD, Yu Z, Sashindranath M, Betz-Stablein B, et al. Assessing the generalizability of deep learning models trained on standardized and nonstandardized images and their performance against Teledermatologists: retrospective comparative study. JMIR Dermatol. 2022;5(3):e35150.
35. Whang SE, Roh Y, Song H, Lee J-G. Data collection and quality challenges in deep learning: a data-centric AI perspective. VLDB J. 2023;32(4):791–813.
36. Willemink MJ, Koszek WA, Hardell C, Wu J, Fleischmann D, Harvey H, et al. Preparing medical imaging data for machine learning. Radiology. 2020;295(1):4–15.
37. Park AJ, Ko JM, Swerlick RA. Crowdsourcing dermatology: DataDerm, big data analytics, and machine learning technology. J Am Acad Dermatol. 2018;78(3):643–4.
38. Yap J, Yolland W, Tschandl P. Multimodal skin lesion classification using deep learning. Exp Dermatol. 2018;27(11):1261–7.
39. Narla S, Heath CR, Alexis A, Silverberg JI. Racial disparities in dermatology. Arch Dermatol Res. 2023;315(5):1215–23.
40. Buster KJ, Stevens EI, Elmets CA. Dermatologic health disparities. Dermatol Clin. 2012;30(1):53–9.
41. Wesley NO, Maibach HI. Racial (ethnic) differences in skin properties: the objective data. Am J Clin Dermatol. 2003;4:843–60.
42. Fliorent R, Fardman B, Podwojniak A, Javaid K, Tan IJ, Ghani H, et al. Artificial intelligence in dermatology: advancements and challenges in skin of color. Int J Dermatol. 2024;63(4):455–61.
43. Pandya AG, Alexis AF, Berger TG, Wintroub BU. Increasing racial and ethnic diversity in dermatology: a call to action. J Am Acad Dermatol. 2016;74(3):584–7.

5 Artificial Intelligence in Predicting Skin-Sensitizing Substances

Karthi Kishore, Siva Chaitanya Senapathi, and Esraa M. AlEdani

5.1 Introduction

Skin sensitization refers to skin exposure to haptens/specific molecules that covalently bind to endogenous proteins due to the electrophilic nature of the chemicals. The process is divided into sensitization and elicitation phases. In sensitization phase, the chemical agent reacts with skin proteins, and dendritic cells process the modified proteins and present the antigen to naive T cells in the local lymph nodes, leading to expansion of antigen-specific T-cell clones. In elicitation phase, subsequent exposure to the same sensitizer elicits a specific T-cell-mediated immune response [1] (Fig. 5.1).

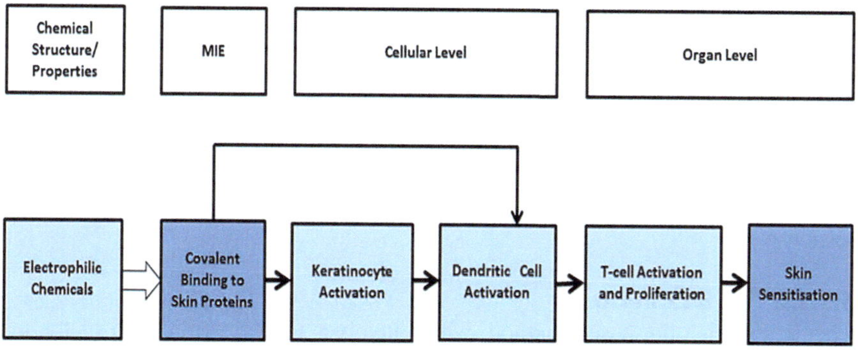

Fig. 5.1 Adverse outcome pathway in case of skin sensitization

K. Kishore (✉) · S. C. Senapathi
Military Hospital Shillong, Shillong, Meghalaya, India

E. M. AlEdani
University of Basrah, College of Medicine, Basra, Iraq

E. M. AlEdani, H. I. Maibach (eds.), *Applications of Artificial Intelligence in Common Dermatological Diseases*, Updates in Clinical Dermatology,
https://doi.org/10.1007/978-3-031-78139-1_5

5.2 Importance of Predicting Skin Sensitization

The prediction of skin sensitization is very essential to identify the hazardous potential of any substance to human health on topical application or ingestion. This is of paramount importance during research development for new drugs, cosmetics, etc. To minimize the occurrence of allergic contact dermatitis (ACD) from exposure to chemical products, national and international regulatory authorities require that skin-sensitizing substances be labelled to identify the potential hazard posed by these items. Such hazards have historically been characterized based on results from animal tests that can use large numbers of animals and produce a painful allergic reaction during testing [2]. Traditionally, the skin sensitization potential of substances has been assessed by using animal models, ranging from guinea pig models to the murine local lymph node assay (LLNA), where the induction phase of the response is quantified by measuring lymphocyte proliferation as a predictive biomarker of skin sensitization. In addition, it measures the estimation concentration (EC3) level, which refers to the test substance concentration inducing a threefold proliferation compared to concurrent vehicle-treated controls, which is inversely proportional to the potency of a skin sensitizer.

5.3 Various Methods Used in Skin Sensitization

5.3.1 Traditional Methods (In Vivo)

5.3.1.1 The Guinea Pig Maximization Test (GPMT)

This is one of the earliest and most widely used methods for evaluating skin sensitization. Developed by Magnusson and Kligman in the 1960s, this method involves both intradermal injection and topical application of a test substance to guinea pigs. The test is divided into induction and challenge phases. During the induction phase, the animals are exposed to the test substance to sensitize them, followed by a rest period. In the challenge phase, the substance is reapplied to assess the sensitization response.

5.3.1.2 The Buehler Test

This is a guinea pig-based method, which involves topical application of the test substance without the need for intradermal injection. This test is generally less invasive and involves fewer procedural steps than the GPMT. This test focuses on repeated application to a single site on the skin, followed by a challenge phase to detect sensitization.

5.3.1.3 The Mouse Local Lymph Node Assay (LLNA)

The local lymph node assay (LLNA) represents a significant advancement over guinea pig models, offering a more refined and ethical approach. Developed in the

1990s, LLNA measures the proliferation of lymphocytes in the lymph nodes draining the site of chemical application on mice. This method provides quantitative data on the sensitizing potential of a substance and is considered less stressful for the animals compared to traditional guinea pig tests.

5.3.1.4 Human Repeated Insult Patch Test (HRIPT)

It is a clinical method that assesses the sensitization potential of a substance through repeated application. This test involves an induction phase, where the substance is applied several times over a few weeks, followed by a challenge phase after a rest period to evaluate any allergic response. RIPT is widely used in the cosmetic and personal care industry to ensure the safety of products.

5.3.2 Drawbacks of Traditional Methods

1. Ethical concerns
2. Limited relevance of animal skin with respect to human skin
3. Time consuming
4. Difficulty in reproducibility
5. Regulatory pressure for alternative methods

5.3.3 Non-animal Models

5.3.3.1 In Vitro Method

This method involves the use of a biological system consisting of cells or tissue models such as primary cultures, finite cell lines, continuous cell lines or reconstructed 3D tissues. The system is based on creating a tissue microenvironment to study the immune response. There is a new concept of OcCs which emphasizes on simulating the structure and physiological properties of tissues or organs, e.g. KeratinoSens, h-CLAT, IL-8 Luc assay [9].

5.3.3.2 Ex Vivo Methods (Isolated Animal Tissues and Organs)

This method uses rat skin transcutaneous electrical resistance (TER) test (OECD TG 430) to assess sensitization. In this technique, skin fragments obtained from humanely euthanized rats is used. The tissue slices from rodents and humans are other alternatives which are used.

5.3.3.3 In Chemico Methods

This comprises various methods that involve the interaction between the test and biological substance, where the resultant reaction is studied, e.g., direct peptide reactivity assay (DPRA).

Direct Peptide Reactivity Assay (DPRA)

The mechanism of this method is to assess a chemical's reactivity against synthetic peptides that have residues of cysteine and lysine. High-performance liquid chromatography is used to quantify the degree of peptide depletion following exposure to a test chemical (HPLC) [10].

5.3.3.4 In Silico Methods

In silico methods involve the use of computational approaches to predict toxicity. It has gained significant attention due to their potential to reduce the need for animal testing and expedite the risk assessment process. The various in silico models used in predicting skin sensitization are as follows:

5.3.3.4.1 Derek Nexus [Detective Estimation of Risk from Existing Knowledge Nexus]

It is an expert system that uses a rule-based approach to predict skin sensitization. It relies on a database of various chemically active groups to determine their sensitization potential. This software applies a rule-based system and knowledge-based algorithms to predict the likelihood of a compound causing an allergic skin reaction (Fig. 5.2).

The Derek Nexus helps to predict skin sensitization in the following ways:

(a) *Structural Alert Identification*: Derek Nexus uses a comprehensive database of structural alerts (chemical substructures) associated with skin sensitization. These alerts are derived from empirical data, including human, animal and in vitro studies. While analysing a chemical structure, Derek Nexus searches for these known sensitizing fragments.
(b) *Mechanistic Understanding*: The software incorporates mechanistic knowledge of skin sensitization, which typically involves a multistep process (Fig. 5.3):

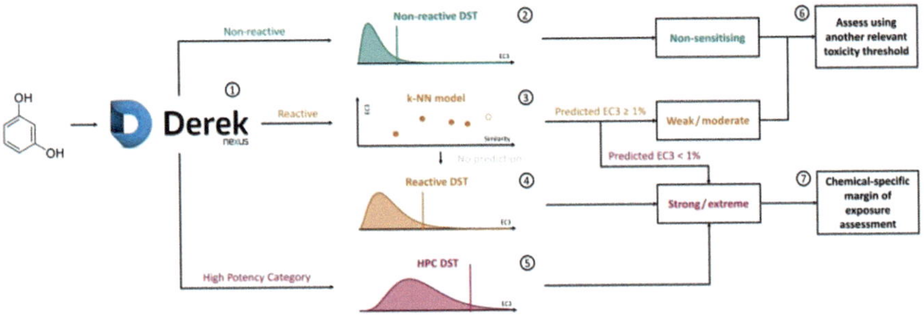

Fig. 5.2 The outline of in silico workflow in Derek Nexus for predicting the skin sensitization potential of various substances

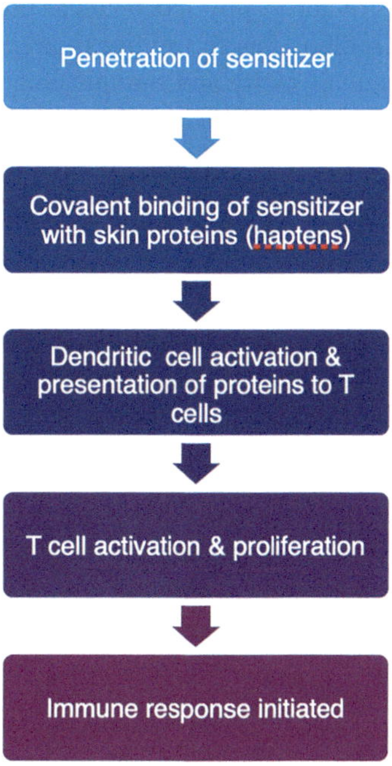

Fig. 5.3 Steps of skin sensitization incorporated in Derek Nexus software

(c) *Rule-Based Reasoning*: Derek Nexus uses rule-based reasoning to predict sensitization potential. It applies a set of predefined rules to determine the likelihood of sensitization based on the presence of specific structural alerts and their known reactivity mechanisms. This reasoning is enhanced by expert knowledge embedded in the system.
(d) *Expert Review and Weight of Evidence*: The predictions made by Derek Nexus are accompanied by a confidence score and an explanation based on the weight of evidence approach. This approach considers the presence of multiple structural alerts, historical data and the reliability of the data sources.
(e) *Integration with Other Tools*: Derek Nexus often integrates with other computational tools and databases, such as Quantitative Structure-Activity Relationship (QSAR) models and the OECD QSAR Toolbox, to provide a more comprehensive assessment [11–15].

The Derek Nexus has 71% accuracy, 53% sensitivity and 76% specificity [16].

5.3.3.4.2 OECD QSAR Toolbox

It is a software application that correlates the chemical structure of substances with their biological activity or properties. The OECD QSAR Toolbox harnesses the power of computational models to predict the potential toxicity, environmental impact and behaviour of chemicals [17]. It integrates a vast database of chemical structures, physicochemical properties and toxicological data. The OECD QSAR Toolbox has the ability to predict endpoints such as acute toxicity, skin irritation, mutagenicity and carcinogenicity of a substance [18]. The Toolbox is an 'all inclusive' tool for the application of category approaches, such as read-across and trend analysis in a single software application. The Toolbox incorporates theoretical knowledge, experimental data and computational tools from various sources into a logical workflow (Fig. 5.4).

The main steps of this workflow are substance identification, identification of relevant structural characteristics and potential toxic mechanisms of interaction, identification of other chemicals having the same structural characteristics and/or mechanism, data collection for the chemicals in the category and use of the existing experimental data to fill the data gap(s). The major functionalities involved in the workflow system of the toolbar are the following:

1. *Input of the Target Substance*
   The data about the various sensitizing substances is fed into the application based on their chemical structure, predefined list of chemicals/inventory/database, drawing of their structure or chemical nomenclature.

2. *Profiling*
   The Profiling module is mainly developed to analyse the target chemical from various aspects such as its reactivity, potency to damage macromolecules, possible interaction mechanisms with receptors, etc. This enables to guide the user towards

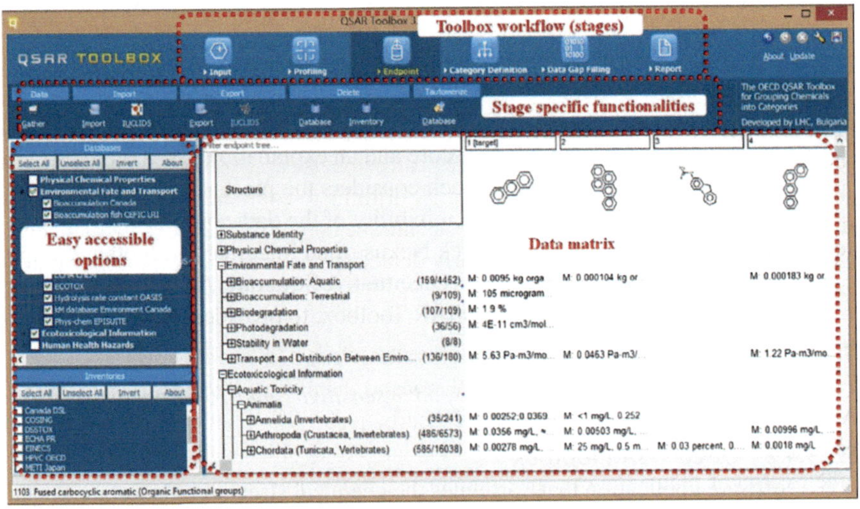

Fig. 5.4 The various components of QSAR OECD Toolbox user interface: workflow steps, step-specific functionalities, easily accessible options and data matrix. (Image source: Dimitrov et al. [19])

the subsequent steps of the workflow. The profile is built based on the following characteristics: structural, functional properties, etc. A set of defined profilers are in the module which is analysing the substance in question. The various profilers in the Toolbox are separated into groups depending on the information they are providing:

(a) Affiliation profilers determine the substance affiliation with databases and inventories.
(b) Generic profilers determine predominantly (bio)chemical properties of the substance that trigger various adverse effects.
(c) Endpoint specific profilers determine substance properties that are related to specific adverse effects such as acute oral toxicity, bioaccumulation or mutagenicity.
(d) Empirical profilers provide basic chemical information such as chemical elements or organic functional groups constituting the substance.
(e) Custom profilers are user-built profilers reflecting the knowledge and experience of users.

These profilers help in the customized categorization of the substances into various groups.

3. *Endpoint Data Collection*

The Endpoint module operates as an information system that changes 'data' into 'information' using processes such as organization, structuring, conversion and modelling of data. In this module data conversion happens which transforms data into meaningful interpretations to improve the user's knowledge and effectiveness of decision-making. The database engine of the *Endpoint* module allows custom databases to be imported into the Toolbox.

4. *Category Definition*

This module provides the user with a means for grouping chemicals into a meaningful category based on their similarity with the target substance. Similarity is not only restricted to structural similarity but also to physical chemical properties, mechanism of interaction, reactive potency or toxicological effects. The chemicals which are similar with respect to skin sensitization which is driven by protein reactivity can be dissimilar with respect to effects such as endocrine disruption which are often driven by non-covalent receptor-mediated interactions. Category definition is the critical step in the workflow of the Toolbox. The stepwise category building results in identification and collection of the most appropriate analogues. It helps in the study of the causality between molecular features and the studied adverse effect/reaction. The process occurs in multiple phases such as initial phase consisting of a lesser conservative collection of an initial group of analogues followed by endpoint specific subcategorization finally resulting in elimination of dissimilar compounds.

5. *Data Gap Filling*

Data gap filling is the process of estimating the property of a non-tested member of a category using the test results available for other members of the category. The Toolbox offers two approaches to predict the target's hazard: read-across and trend analysis. In addition, the Toolbox has a library of independent QSAR models that can be applied to the target chemical. The Toolbox provides a variety of formal, statistical and logical approaches to analyse systematically the data pattern. Among the formal tools are data transformation, data filtering by test conditions, depicting details for a substance, etc.

6. *Reporting*

Three types of reports approved by the OECD and ECHA are produced by the Toolbox:

(i) *Chemical Category Reporting Format (CCRF)*

CCRF is based on the OECD's Guidance on Grouping of Chemicals, where information about a particular category is summarized based on its scientific rationale, domain, associated endpoints, the members of the category as well as the justification for the robustness of the category.

(ii) *Toolbox Prediction Reporting Format (TPRF)*

TPRF is based on the QSAR Prediction Reporting Format created by the European Chemicals Bureau and was modified to accommodate the functionalities of the Toolbox.

(iii) *Toolbox Model Reporting Format (TMRF)*

TMRF is based on the QSAR Model Reporting Format (QMRF) version created by the European Chemicals Bureau and was modified to accommodate the functionalities of the OECD Toolbox [19]. The OECD QSAR model has lower accuracy (48%), higher sensitivity (100%) and lower specificity (0%) compared to in vivo test [20].

5.3.3.4.3 TOPKAT

TOPKAT (Toxicity Prediction by Komputer Assisted Technology) is a computational tool that uses QSAR models to predict various toxicological endpoints, including skin sensitization where statistical models from a large dataset of chemical structures and their biological activities are employed [21]. The functioning of TOPKAT which predicts skin sensitization involves several key steps, grounded in computational toxicology and chemoinformatics:

1. *Database of Known Toxicants*: TOPKAT relies on a curated database of chemicals with known toxicological profiles. This database includes extensive experimental data on skin sensitization, which serves as the reference set.
2. *Molecular Descriptors*: The software calculates molecular descriptors for each chemical. These descriptors are quantitative representations of molecular prop-

erties, such as hydrophobicity, electronic distribution, molecular shape and hydrogen bonding potential. They are essential in capturing the chemical features relevant to skin sensitization.

3. *Quantitative Structure-Activity Relationship (QSAR) Models*: TOPKAT employs QSAR models, which correlate molecular descriptors with biological activity. These models are generated using statistical and machine learning techniques, such as regression analysis and neural networks, trained on the experimental data from the database. QSAR models predict the likelihood that a chemical will cause skin sensitization based on its molecular structure.
4. *Validation and Verification*: The QSAR models in TOPKAT undergo rigorous validation and verification processes to ensure their accuracy and reliability. This involves dividing the dataset into training and test sets, cross-validation and external validation using independent datasets.
5. *Prediction*: When a new chemical is analysed, TOPKAT calculates its molecular descriptors and applies the QSAR models to predict its potential for skin sensitization. The prediction is usually accompanied by a confidence level, reflecting the model's certainty in its assessment [22–24].

5.3.3.4.4 TIMES-SS (Tissue Metabolism Simulator for Skin Sensitization)

It refers to a mechanistic model that simulates the metabolic activation of chemicals to study their subsequent interaction with skin proteins and thereby assess their sensitization potential [25].

The mechanisms of TIMES-SS are as follows:

1. *Metabolic Simulation*

TIMES-SS predicts the metabolic fate of chemicals by simulating phase I and phase II metabolic reactions, which identifies the reactive metabolites which act as skin sensitizers. These simulations help in identifying the formation of reactive metabolites which could act as skin sensitizers.

2. *Electrophilic Reactivity*

The model evaluates the potential of chemicals and their metabolites to form covalent bonds with skin proteins, a key step in the skin sensitization process. It focuses on the ability of chemicals to act as electrophiles and form haptens that bind to skin proteins.

3. *Quantitative Structure-Activity Relationship (QSAR)*

QSAR models are employed to predict the sensitization potential based on the structural properties of chemicals. The TIMES-SS uses a database of known sensitizers to train its algorithms and improve prediction accuracy.

4. *Mechanistic Domains*

TIMES-SS classifies chemicals into different mechanistic domains based on their structural alerts and reactivity profiles. These domains help in understanding the specific pathways through which a chemical might act as a sensitizer.

5. *Local Lymph Node Assay (LLNA) Correlation*
   The model's predictions are often correlated with LLNA data, a standard in vivo test for skin sensitization. This helps in validating the predictive performance of TIMES-SS [26–28]. The TIME SS has 67% accuracy, 55% sensitivity and 71% specificity [16].

5.3.3.4.5 Tox21

The aim of the 'Toxicity Testing in the Twenty-First Century' (Tox21) initiative was to develop more efficient and less time-consuming approaches to predicting how chemicals affect human health [29, 30]. It aims at employing computational methods to screen large number of compounds over a short span of time [31]. The computational methods in order to be universally validated must achieve comparable results with respect to traditional biological experiments. The aim of Tox21 Challenge was to assess the above-mentioned, where various participants were invited to develop various computational methods to predict the toxic potential of compounds. The training set consisted of the Tox21 10K compound library, which includes environmental chemicals and drugs. The toxicity prediction of compounds was done using machine learning methods, where the chemical compounds are represented by chemical descriptors which are fed into a predictor. Methods for predicting biological effects are usually categorized into similarity-based approaches and feature-based approaches. Similarity-based methods compute a matrix of pairwise similarities between compounds which is subsequently used by the prediction algorithms [32].

The Tox21 Challenge unfolded in several key phases, each with distinct goals and datasets:

1. *Data Preprocessing and Baseline Models*: Participants were first tasked with preprocessing the provided datasets and developing baseline predictive models. This phase emphasized the importance of data quality and feature selection in building robust models.
2. *Model Development and Optimization*: The main phase of the challenge involved developing and optimizing machine learning models to predict the toxicity of unknown chemicals. Various techniques, including neural networks, support vector machines and ensemble methods, were employed by participants.
3. *Evaluation and Validation*: The final phase focused on evaluating the performance of submitted models using an independent test set. The models were assessed based on their predictive accuracy, robustness and generalizability.

5.3.4 Deep Learning Models/Deep Neural Network

Deep neural networks (DNNs) comprise many hidden layers with a great number of neurons. A DNN may have thousands of neurons in each layer, which is in contrast to traditional artificial neural networks that employ only a small number of neurons. The goal is no longer to just learn the main pieces of information, but rather to capture all possible facets of the input. Deep learning was applied to predict the outcome of biological assays which made it a prime candidate for toxicity prediction [33]. In each layer deep learning constructs features in neurons that are connected to neurons of the previous layer. Thus, the input data is represented by features in each layer, where features in higher layers code more abstract input concepts [34]. The availability of high-throughput toxicity assays provides sufficient data to use deep learning for toxicity prediction [29, 30].

5.3.4.1 DeepTox

DeepTox is a deep learning model designed to predict the toxicity of chemical compounds, including their potential to cause skin sensitization. It leverages large datasets and advanced neural network architectures to improve the accuracy of toxicity predictions. Here's a detailed overview of its performance and application in predicting skin sensitization, supported by scientific references:

5.3.4.1.1 Overview of DeepTox

1. *Deep Learning Model*: DeepTox utilizes deep neural networks, which are capable of capturing complex patterns in data. This makes them particularly suited for toxicity prediction tasks where traditional methods might fall short.
2. *Training Data*: The model is trained on large datasets of chemical compounds and their known toxicological outcomes. For skin sensitization, it typically uses data from sources like the database of Quantitative Structure-Activity Relationships (QSAR), public toxicity databases and proprietary datasets from chemical companies.
3. *Descriptors*: DeepTox employs molecular descriptors and fingerprints that encode the structural information of chemical compounds. These descriptors are crucial for the model to learn the relationship between chemical structure and toxicological outcome.

5.3.4.1.2 Performance in Predicting Skin Sensitization

1. *Accuracy*: Studies have shown that DeepTox can achieve high accuracy in predicting skin sensitization. For example, one study reported that DeepTox achieved an accuracy of over 80% in predicting skin sensitization, outperforming several traditional QSAR models.
2. *Validation*: The performance of DeepTox has been validated using various datasets, including the Interagency Coordinating Committee on the Validation of Alternative Methods (ICCVAM) dataset for skin sensitization. Validation studies demonstrate that DeepTox has a high sensitivity and specificity, indicating its reliability in predicting true positives and true negatives in skin sensitization.
3. *Benchmarking*: DeepTox has been benchmarked against other computational models and has shown superior performance in many cases. For instance, a com-

parative study showed that DeepTox outperformed other machine learning models, such as random forests and support vector machines, in predicting the skin sensitization potential of chemicals.

5.3.4.1.3 Applications and Implications

1. *Regulatory Use*: DeepTox's ability to accurately predict skin sensitization has significant implications for regulatory toxicology. It can be used as a part of an integrated testing strategy (ITS) to reduce the need for animal testing, in line with the principles of the 3Rs (Replacement, Reduction, Refinement).
2. *Chemical Safety*: By predicting the skin sensitization potential of new and existing chemicals, DeepTox aids in the safety assessment of consumer products, pharmaceuticals and industrial chemicals. This helps in ensuring that only safe products reach the market.
3. *Drug Development*: In the pharmaceutical industry, DeepTox can be used to screen potential drug candidates for skin sensitization early in the development process, thus reducing the risk of adverse effects in later stages of drug development [35–39].

5.3.5 Integrated Models

Though stand-alone methods have demonstrated to be applicable for some specific toxicological predictions with some limitations, the new strategy for the application of newer approaches, to solve complex toxicological endpoints, is addressed by Integrated Approaches for Testing and Assessment (IATA) or Integrated Testing Strategies (ITS). It has been described by OECD as 'pragmatic, science-based approaches for chemical hazard characterization that rely on an integrated analysis of existing information coupled with the generation of new information using testing strategies. IATA follow an iterative approach to answer a defined question in a specific regulatory context, taking into account the acceptable level of uncertainty associated with the decision context'. In this model various in vivo, in silico and in chemico models are combined to achieve most accurate and optimal results/interpretation. The various testing strategies in this model are combined and weighed in a fixed way which would serve to replace some or all of the in vivo methods to predict toxicity endpoints.

The reasons for developing the integrated models are as follows:

(a) To encourage thorough coverage of all possible outcomes.
(b) To reduce the number of false positive and increase positive predictive value.
(c) The gold standard biological tests have various ethical concerns and are labour-intensive, so these models act as a suitable alternative.
(d) To enhance coverage of maximum database available under various domains [40].

5.4 The Applications of AI in Predicting Skin Sensitization

1. *Classification of Skin Sensitizers*

The various algorithms provided by AI models such as support vector machines (SVM), random forests (RF) and neural networks (NN) help in the classification of various substances as sensitizers and non-sensitizers. Quantitative Structure-Activity Relationship (QSAR) model helps predict the skin sensitization potential based on the chemical structure of substances.

2. *Development of Database and AI Model Training*

AI helps in the assimilation of various data available through various in vivo and in vitro models such as direct peptide reactivity assay (DPRA) and human Cell Line Activation Test (h-CLAT) to create algorithm for predicting a substance sensitization. In silico models such as QSAR can be used for analysing skin sensitizers and hence can be used to develop algorithms for determining the potency of skin sensitization.

3. Establishment of Tools for Skin Sensitization

(a) *OECD QSAR Toolbox*

This is a tool that integrates various QSAR models and databases to predict skin sensitization.

(b) *KNIME*

This is an open-source data analytics platform that supports the integration of ML algorithms for toxicological predictions. We have created a KNIME-verified component that flags input molecules upon their potential skin sensitization capability. It is based on 51 revised SMARTS that are documented within the component and accessible to the community. While flagging compounds with toxicological alerts based on their structure is a valuable part of QSAR, thereby contributing to Adverse Outcome pathway (AOPs), their outcome should be taken reasonably. If a chemical fails to trigger any of the electrophilic rules coded in the SMARTS patterns, it does not necessarily mean that it will be a non-sensitizer. The resulting classification should not be used in isolation and is ideally combined with other weighted evidence and information.

5.5 Advantages of AI in Predicting Skin Sensitization

1. *High Accuracy*: AI algorithms can achieve high accuracy in predicting skin sensitization by analysing vast amounts of data, including molecular structures, chemical properties and biological responses.
2. *Efficiency*: AI models can process large datasets and perform complex calculations much faster than traditional methods, reducing time and resources required for prediction.

3. *Identification of New Chemical Entities*: AI can identify potential skin sensitizers among new chemical entities early in the drug development process, helping to prioritize compounds for further testing.

5.6 Disadvantages of AI in Predicting Skin Sensitization

1. *Data Quality*: The accuracy of AI predictions heavily depends on the quality and quantity of input data. Biased or incomplete datasets can lead to inaccurate predictions.
2. *Interpretability*: AI models, especially deep learning algorithms, can be complex and difficult to interpret, making it challenging to understand the reasoning behind specific predictions.
3. *Regulatory Acceptance*: Regulatory agencies may require transparent and interpretable models for risk assessment, which can be a challenge for some AI techniques.
4. *Ethical Concerns*: The use of AI in skin sensitization prediction raises ethical concerns regarding privacy, data security and potential biases in algorithmic decision-making.

5.7 Conclusion

AI plays a crucial role in predicting skin sensitization, a process that involves identifying substances that can cause an allergic reaction upon contact with the skin. Traditional methods of testing for skin sensitization, such as animal testing and human patch testing, are time-consuming, costly and often ethically problematic. AI offers a more efficient and accurate alternative by leveraging large datasets, advanced algorithms and machine learning techniques.

One key application of AI in predicting skin sensitization is through the development of computational models. These models are trained on vast amounts of chemical and biological data to recognize patterns and correlations between chemical structures and their potential to cause skin allergies. By analysing molecular features, such as chemical composition, structure-activity relationships and physicochemical properties, AI algorithms can classify substances as sensitizers or non-sensitizers with high accuracy. Moreover, AI enables the integration of diverse sources of information, including in vitro test results, clinical data and toxicological studies, into predictive models. This multidimensional approach enhances the reliability and robustness of predictions, allowing for comprehensive assessments of skin sensitization potential across various chemical classes and formulations. Furthermore, AI-driven tools facilitate the rapid screening of large chemical libraries, accelerating the identification of potential sensitizers while reducing the need for extensive experimental testing. This not only saves time and resources but also promotes the development of safer and more sustainable products in industries such as cosmetics, pharmaceuticals and chemicals.

AI's predictive capabilities in skin sensitization extend beyond hazard assessment to include risk assessment and personalized medicine. By analysing individual susceptibility factors, such as genetic variations, immune responses and environmental exposures, AI systems can predict an individual's likelihood of developing skin allergies and recommend personalized prevention strategies and treatments.

In conclusion, AI plays a pivotal role in revolutionizing the prediction of skin sensitization by offering faster, more accurate and ethically sound alternatives to traditional testing methods. Its applications span hazard assessment, risk prediction and personalized healthcare, contributing to safer products and improved dermatological outcomes.

References

1. Carney EW, Settivari R. A comprehensive guide to toxicology in preclinical drug development. Academic Press; 2013.
2. Strickland J, Zang Q, Paris M, Lehmann DM, Allen D, Choksi N, Matheson J, Jacobs A, Casey W, Kleinstreuer N. Multivariate models for prediction of human skin sensitization hazard. J Appl Toxicol. 2017;37(3):347–60.
3. Basketter DA, Blaikie L, Dearman RJ, Kimber I, Ryan CA, Gerberick GF, Harvey P, Evans P, White IR, Rycroft RJ. Use of the local lymph node assay for the estimation of relative contact allergenic potency. Contact Derm. 2000;42(6):344–8.
4. Selgrade MK, Sullivan KS, Boyles RR, Dederick E, Serex TL, Loveless SE. Decision trees for evaluating skin and respiratory sensitizing potential of chemicals in accordance with European regulations. Regul Toxicol Pharmacol. 2012;63(3):371–80.
5. Magnusson B, Kligman AM. The identification of contact allergens by animal assay. The Guinea pig maximization test. J Invest Dermatol. 1969;52(3):268–76.
6. Buehler EV. Delayed contact hypersensitivity in the Guinea Pig. Arch Dermatol. 1965;91:171–7.
7. Kimber I, Basketter DA, Gerberick GF, Dearman RJ. The local lymph node assay: a viable alternative to currently accepted skin sensitization tests. Food Chem Toxicol. 1994;32(6):543–7.
8. Marzulli FN, Maibach HI. Contact allergy: predictive testing in humans. Adv Modern Toxicol. 1974;4:353–72.
9. Aleksic M, Rajagopal R, de Ávila R, Spriggs S, Gilmour N. The skin sensitization adverse outcome pathway: exploring the role of mechanistic understanding for higher tier risk assessment. Crit Rev Toxicol. 2024;54(2):69–91.
10. Gerberick GF, Vassallo JD, Bailey RE, Chaney JG, Morrall SW, Lepoittevin JP. Development of a peptide reactivity assay for screening contact allergens. Toxicol Sci. 2007;97(2):417–27.
11. Roberts DW, Aptula AO. Role of hydrophobicity and reactivity in skin sensitization potency of contact allergens. Chem Res Toxicol. 2014;27(6):1191–204.
12. Murphy J, et al. Evaluation of in silico models for skin sensitization. Regul Toxicol Pharmacol. 2019;106:18–26.
13. Takahashi K, et al. Regulatory application of integrated testing strategies for skin sensitization. Toxicol In Vitro. 2019;55:189–97.

14. Hewitt P, et al. Use of in silico systems and expert knowledge in safety assessment. J Appl Toxicol. 2013;33(11):1413–22.
15. Van der Veen J, et al. Predictive models for skin sensitization: performance of Derek Nexus and other tools. Comput Toxicol. 2014;1:12–24.
16. Fitzpatrick JM, Roberts DW, Patlewicz G. An evaluation of selected (Q)SARs/expert systems for predicting skin sensitisation potential. SAR QSAR Environ Res. 2018;29(6):439–68.
17. Organisation for Economic Co-operation and Development (OECD). QSAR Toolbox. Retrieved from OECD QSAR Toolbox Website.
18. Patlewicz G, Jeliazkova N, Safford RJ, Worth AP. A practical guide to QSAR and data mining. In: Silico toxicology: principles and applications. Royal Society of Chemistry; 2008. p. 77–100.
19. Dimitrov SD, Diderich R, Sobanski T, et al. QSAR Toolbox - workflow and major functionalities. SAR QSAR Environ Res. 2016;27(3):203–19. https://doi.org/10.1080/1062936X.2015.1136680.
20. Strickland J, Truax J, Corvaro M, Settivari R, Henriquez J, McFadden J, Gulledge T, Johnson V, Gehen S, Germolec D, Allen DG, Kleinstreuer N. Application of defined approaches for skin sensitization to agrochemical products. Front Toxicol. 2022;4:852856.
21. Enslein K, Blake BW. Use of TOPKAT to predict the carcinogenicity of chemicals. Environ Health Perspect. 1994;102(Suppl 1):109–12.
22. Roberts DW, Patlewicz G. Non-animal skin sensitization methods: advances and challenges. Curr Opin Toxicol. 2018;9:43–7.
23. Helma C. Predictive toxicology. CRC Press; 2006.
24. Patlewicz G, Jeliazkova N, Safford RJ, Worth AP, Aleksiev B. An evaluation of the implementation of the cramer classification scheme in the Toxtree software. SAR QSAR Environ Res. 2008;19(5–6):495–524.
25. Dimitrov SD, Low LK, Patlewicz GY, Kern PS, Dimitrova ND, Comber MH, et al. TIMES--SS–a mechanistic evaluation of an external validation study using reaction chemistry principles. Chem Res Toxicol. 2005;18(7):937–52.
26. Patlewicz G, et al. Can currently available QSAR models be used to support the use of the 'read-across' approach to fill data gaps in skin sensitisation risk assessment? Regul Toxicol Pharmacol. 2014;72(1):116–29.
27. Dimitrov SD, et al. Simulation of chemical metabolism for fate and hazard assessment. III. New developments of the bioconcentration factor base-line model. Chemosphere. 2005;61(11):1570–83.
28. OECD. Guidance document on the use of adverse outcome pathways in developing Integrated Approaches to Testing and Assessment (IATA). Series on Testing and Assessment No. 260. 2016.
29. Andersen ME, Krewski D. Toxicity testing in the 21st century: bringing the vision to life. Toxicol Sci. 2009;107(2):324–30.
30. Krewski D, Acosta D Jr, Andersen M, et al. Toxicity testing in the 21st century: a vision and a strategy. J Toxicol Environ Health B Crit Rev. 2010;13(2–4):51–138.
31. Rusyn I, Daston GP. Computational toxicology: realizing the promise of the toxicity testing in the 21st century. Environ Health Perspect. 2010;118(8):1047–50.
32. Kauffman GW, Jurs PC. QSAR and k-nearest neighbor classification analysis of selective cyclooxygenase-2 inhibitors using topologically-based numerical descriptors. J Chem Inf Comput Sci. 2001;41(6):1553–60.
33. Unterthiner T, Mayr A, Klambauer G, et al. Proceedings of the deep learning workshop at NIPS. Deep learning as an opportunity in virtual screening. 12 Dec 2014.
34. LeCun Y, Bengio Y, Hinton G. Deep learning. Nature. 2015;521:436–44.
35. Mayr A, et al. DeepTox: toxicity prediction using deep learning. Front Environ Sci. 2016;

36. Wang S, et al. Deep learning toxicity prediction: challenges and future directions. J Chem Inf Model. 2018;
37. Hong H, et al. Comparison of deep learning and traditional machine learning approaches for QSAR modeling of environmental chemicals. Chemosphere. 2017;
38. Gupta R, et al. Evaluation of DeepTox in predicting chemical toxicity. Regul Toxicol Pharmacol. 2019;
39. Thomas RS, et al. Use of deep learning models for regulatory toxicology applications. Comput Toxicol. 2019;
40. Hartung T, Luechtefeld T, Maertens A, et al. Integrated testing strategies for safety assessments. ALTEX. 2013;30:3–18.

Limitations and Challenges of AI in Dermatology

6

Esraa M. AlEdani

6.1 Overview

In dermatology, artificial intelligence (AI) based on convolutional neural networks (CNNs) and machine learning (ML) is quickly becoming a viable possibility. While melanoma is one of the deadliest types of cancer, non-melanoma skin cancer is the most frequent type of cancer in the world. Dermoscopy has increased doctors' diagnostic precision in identifying skin cancer, but sadly, it is still quite low.

AI may be of great use in the early detection and diagnosis of skin cancer. The previous 10 years have seen significant advancements in the field of artificial intelligence, having performance that is better than or at least on par with clinicians. While several studies have demonstrated highly promising findings for skin cancer diagnosis using AI algorithms, their generalizability and practicality in routine clinical practice are yet unknown.

Here, we tried to highlight the possible drawbacks and difficulties with AI that were highlighted in various studies and identify solutions to overcome these obstacles in next research. Lastly, we attempted to examine the benefits and prospects that the possible application of AI in dermatology procedures might bring about for patients and the field as a whole.

6.2 Pitfalls in AI

At this time, it's important to recognize the potential drawbacks of AI as well as its benefits and future prospects. Numerous research studies have demonstrated that the existence of confounding factors can have a negative effect on AI systems'

E. M. AlEdani (✉)
University of Basrah, College of Medicine, Basra, Iraq

E. M. AlEdani, H. I. Maibach (eds.), *Applications of Artificial Intelligence in Common Dermatological Diseases*, Updates in Clinical Dermatology,
https://doi.org/10.1007/978-3-031-78139-1_6

categorization ability. These elements are primarily related to standardization and picture quality characteristics. Variables that rely on the quality of the image provided by a clinician include image rotation, adversarial "noise" (intended perturbations like ink spots intended to "confuse" MLA), rulers, brightness/contrast manipulation, ink markings, blurry photos, and dark corners of the tubular lens.

According to a study, the AI algorithm seems to have a higher likelihood of interpreting photos. Right now, we must recognize the possible drawbacks of AI while also pointing out its benefits and future prospects. Numerous research studies have demonstrated that confounding circumstances can have a negative effect on the categorization performance of AI systems. These elements mostly relate to image quality and standardization variables. The quality of an image provided by a clinician determines a number of variables, including image rotation, adversarial "noise" (intended perturbations like ink spots intended to "confuse" MLA), brightness/contrast manipulation, rulers, ink markings, blurry photos, and dark corners of the tubular lens.

In particular, a study found that the AI system seemed more likely to interpret images. Additionally, the ISIC Archive and artificial intelligence researchers have noted that the majority of patients in training datasets for AI algorithms are Caucasian, which may limit the representation of potential variation in disease presentation. Furthermore, compared to common distributions, a study showed that less accurate classifications by the algorithms were produced by rarer distributions of particular skin lesions, such as nonpigmented nevi and nonpigmented MMs. These findings demonstrate the need to evaluate algorithms on both common and uncommon types of lesions and imaging characteristics.

In order to display the lesion under examination in a more realistic and accurate manner, further study is required on the combination of clinical close-up images with dermoscopic images as specified by combined convolutional neural networks (cCNNs). These up-close photos may offer more datasets for upcoming artificial intelligence preclinical assessments. All things considered, deep learning is a very data-intensive technology that needs a large amount of labeled samples in order to accomplish correct classification. Since machine learning (ML) is only as good as the quality of the data it receives, ISIC is the beginning of a publicly accessible image dataset that needs to grow with the collaborative approach of frontline clinicians in order to design and train classifiers with the best outcomes.

6.3 Hurdles to Implementation

Many obstacles related to technology, medical practice foundations, and accessibility have caused the use of AI in dermatology offices to proceed slowly. Notwithstanding the many benefits that come with integrating AI into the healthcare industry, there are some obstacles that need to be solved. Ethical and legal concerns surrounding the development and acquisition of AI learning models are among these obstacles. Healthcare providers must adhere to stringent regulations, including not disclosing patient information to third parties, in order to comply with laws protecting patient confidentiality in healthcare, such as the Health Insurance Portability and Accountability Act of 1996 (HIPAA).

This has shown to be a barrier to accessing a large amount of healthcare data for AI developers. Additionally, this restriction might have an impact on the variety of datasets and images that these AI systems process, which could have a detrimental effect on healthcare disparities and increase their prevalence. In areas with various ethnic backgrounds, the application of models derived from non-inclusive global databases may lead to inaccurate patient diagnoses. Furthermore, there is a lot of variation in how the same diseases manifest in different groups. Preventing incorrect diagnoses of individuals is crucial, particularly for Black, Indigenous, and People of Color (BIPOC) groups.

For instance, psoriasis in black people usually manifests as violet with an ash-gray scale, whereas in white people, it usually manifests as red or pink with a silvery scale. Similarities to this phenomenon may be seen in cellulitis, vitiligo, eczema, and melanoma.

One way to address this issue is to highlight a vast and comprehensive image library that covers a range of skin tones. Data from racially and ethnically diverse groups may also be obtained and may be helpful. One such clinical system support program that tries to assist medical professionals in their differential diagnosis is called VisualDx. It makes use of desktop and mobile apps to help identify patient patterns of skin symptoms. Frequent testing of AI software and the organic advancement of technology offer further solutions to this problem. A dermatologist then needs to collect biographical and medical data with the skin scans in order to accurately deliver a comprehensive diagnosis.

In other words, a dermatologist can't create a treatment plan using just a portion of the patient's data; technology must advance to combine clinical information with skin scans. The application of AI will cause a significant change in dermatology; most notably, the knowledge and capacity to identify melanoma early on will be essential to propelling AI to the forefront of cancer treatment across all specialties. Because AI will be directly responsible for extending medical education and producing new jobs in the health business, it will transform both medical treatment and the workforce as a whole. In the same way that no one will be able to handle AI technology, only specialists in computer science, like data architects, will possess the training needed to expand, create, and store the data that AI algorithms need.

The healthcare team will also need to be exposed to more clinical data; as AI becomes a more tangible and significant component of clinical decision-making, doctors, nurses, and physician assistants will need to complete further medical education in the field. In order to better prepare new doctors or data scientists for the healthcare industry's technological demands, there has been a push recently in European countries for dual degrees that mix science and technology. All things considered, the need for technological innovations to address the issues of patient volume, aging, and effective care is causing rapid shifts in the healthcare workforce.

6.4 Clinical Limitations in AI

Clinical evaluation, comprising patient history and examination, is the foundation for all physicians. In the artificial circumstances of tasks and studies to measure CNN performance, the clinician's skill is frequently underestimated. Many studies acknowledge the absence of clinically relevant variables such as age, gender, degree of sun exposure, anatomic site, and personal and family history. In a clinical setting, dermatologists would perform a total body examination to compare variables such as the macroscopic Ugly Duckling sign (a nevus that stands out from the rest in a given individual), the Little Red Riding Hood sign (a nevus that appears benign but differs from the rest in a given individual), and dermatoscopic predominant nevus patterns (defined as the pattern seen in more than 30% of all nevi).

These approaches improve sensitivity and specificity but necessitate a more comprehensive approach. Furthermore, an experimental design showed that in vivo dermoscopy is intrinsically superior to an artificial environment based only on digital images. Consumer trust in AI is another hurdle to AI's use in healthcare practice. A recent study attempted to shed light on citizens' trust and expectations for the deployment of AI across several countries. Researchers found that the adequacy of current regulations and legislations for the safe use of AI is the most powerful motivator for their trust. Furthermore, 63% of respondents reported being unwilling or uncertain about trusting AI in healthcare. The black box character of ML stems from the lack of a clear explanation and consistent methodology for how the algorithm arrived at a certain diagnosis. This technique may cause patients to lose faith, especially if the model provides a diagnostic output but does not explain the results. Physician interpretation is required to explain why a particular diagnosis or treatment should be chosen. As previously indicated, TBSE is not yet widely available to patients. According to studies, primary care physicians (PCPs) and dermatologists rarely perform TBSE as part of their routine practice assessment. Despite the fact that the significance of TBSE has been highlighted in numerous research, there are no universal guidelines among specialists on skin cancer screening to ensure the use of this diagnostic method. Furthermore, limited time and training for medical students and residents precludes TBSE from being used in clinical practice. The application of AI in TBSE could be a useful helper to PCPs and other non-dermatology specialists, as it will give patients with skin cancer screenings that they would not otherwise receive, while saving physicians' time. Even the best algorithm or clinician will be unable to diagnose an unexamined or unimaged melanoma; thus our efforts should surely be concentrated in this area. Finally, we don't know whether all of these efforts to detect skin cancer early on are beneficial or dangerous.

Overdiagnosis is a common word used to describe a wide range of illnesses, some of which have unclear biology. Within that continuum, we are unsure if excessive usage of technology can deviate from the anticipated outcomes. The dilemma revolves around two key concerns: the discovery of melanocytic tumors at an exceedingly early stage with unclear malignant potential and the over-detection of Non-melanoma skin cancer (NMSC) in elderly patients. This can have a negative psychological impact on patients in the early stages of MM, as well as redundant excisions for NMSC in patients with a short life expectancy, casting doubt on the value of such excisions.

6.5 How to Overcome Limitations

There are potential solutions to these flaws before these algorithms become a part of daily therapeutic practice. First, we must extend CNN training sets to match the diversity of the general population. The immigrant waves underpin this need since physicians are compelled to examine patient populations with which they are unfamiliar and have less to appraise. A trained algorithm will thus provide an advantage. Most algorithms are developed on Caucasian or Asian patients, although early screening of people with skin of color may be more useful, as delayed diagnosis has been associated with more severe disease and shorter survival rates in this population. Metadata for the patients being examined, such as age, gender, skin type, and anatomic location, should become an inseparable component of the data presented to the algorithm. This will create a more realistic study environment for professionals who always use a patient's history in their diagnostic approach. Future research will determine whether this approach provides clinicians with better accuracy than CNNs. Clinical close-up photos can also be used to artificially classify skin lesions. A clinician's initial step in determining whether or not to proceed with dermoscopy is to examine a lesion macroscopically. Clinical pictures of the lesion can reveal additional data that dermoscopy cannot, such as the pearly appearance and shiny surface of BCC and the "stuck-on" appearance of seborrheic keratosis. The combination of clinical and dermoscopic image analysis is known as combined CNN (cCNN), and it is likely to become the standard reference point in future investigations. Previous research has used cCNN classifiers to improve algorithm performance. A variety of strategies for lesion segmentation have been proposed and may be employed in future investigations. A study found that the overall performance of lesion classifiers trained on segmented pictures was comparable to that of unsegmented ones. However, researchers emphasized that segmentation quality must be monitored, as this approach may present new dangers that necessitate additional research. Finally, rather than viewing human and artificial intelligence as adversaries in reader studies, the scientific community should support studies that promote collaboration. In Hekler et al.'s investigation, dermatologists and a single trained CNN classifier independently diagnosed a set of biopsy-verified skin lesions. The researchers pooled their findings to create a new ensemble classifier with increased sensitivity compared to the best individual classifier.

References

1. Liopyris K, Gregoriou S, Dias J, et al. Artificial intelligence in dermatology: challenges and perspectives. Dermatol Ther (Heidelb). 2022;12:2637–51. https://doi.org/10.1007/s13555-022-00833-8.

2. Sathe A, Seth I, Bulloch G, Xie Y, Hunter-Smith DJ, Rozen WM. The role of artificial intelligence language models in dermatology: opportunities, limitations and ethical considerations. Australas J Dermatol. 2023;64(4):548–52. https://doi.org/10.1111/ajd.14133. Epub 2023 Jul 21. PMID: 37477340
3. Koka SS, Burkhart CG. Artificial intelligence in dermatology: current uses, shortfalls, and potential opportunities for further implementation in diagnostics and care. Open Dermatol J. 2023;17(1)

7 Ethical, Legal, and Practical Considerations

Esraa M. AlEdani

7.1 Bias and Fairness in AI Dermatology Tools

7.1.1 Introduction

Disparities in healthcare results can be due to bias in AI systems, especially in fields like dermatology where visual analysis is essential. Large datasets are essential for training dermatological AI technologies, particularly those built on deep learning. The models might perform poorly for some populations, especially those with darker skin tones, if these datasets are not representative of the larger patient population [1].

7.1.2 Sources of Bias

- *Data Imbalance:* Due to historical and regional biases in data collection, a large number of dermatological datasets are biased toward lighter skin tones.
- *Labeling Errors:* Training can be hampered by inaccurate or inconsistent skin condition labeling, which disproportionately affects less frequent presentations.
- *Algorithmic Bias:* Model architectures and training protocols have the potential to perpetuate existing inequities, even in the case of balanced datasets [1].

E. M. AlEdani (✉)
University of Basrah, College of Medicine, Basra, Iraq

E. M. AlEdani, H. I. Maibach (eds.), *Applications of Artificial Intelligence in Common Dermatological Diseases*, Updates in Clinical Dermatology,
https://doi.org/10.1007/978-3-031-78139-1_7

7.1.3 Case Study

According to a 2019 study, patients with Fitzpatrick skin types V and VI had far lower melanoma diagnosis accuracy when using numerous AI dermatology techniques.

Concerns regarding unequal care have been raised by commercial applications' failure to identify significant skin problems in persons of color.

7.1.4 Mitigation Strategies

Diverse Data Collection: Working together with organizations throughout the world to produce inclusive datasets.

Regular assessments of model performance across demographic subgroups are known as *bias audits.*

Fairness-Aware Algorithms: Equitable performance measurements are achieved by incorporating fairness requirements during training [1].

7.2 Regulatory Challenges and Clinical Validation

7.2.1 Regulatory Frameworks

Regulatory bodies like the European Medicines Agency (EMA) and the US Food and Drug Administration (FDA) frequently classify AI tools in dermatology, especially diagnostic systems, as medical devices. Strict safety, effectiveness, and transparency standards are imposed by this categorization [2].

7.2.2 Challenges in Regulation

Adaptive Algorithms: Conventional validation frameworks are made more difficult by certain AI models that keep learning after deployment.

Transparency: Since deep learning models are frequently regarded as "black boxes," it is challenging to explain the reasoning behind judgments, which is a major regulatory concern.

Clinical Trial Design: New trial designs that take into consideration real-world application and human-AI collaboration are necessary for validating AI solutions [2].

7.2.3 Emerging Approaches

Total Product Lifecycle (TPLC): The FDA's suggested TPLC strategy places a strong emphasis on ongoing supervision, which includes performance monitoring in the real world.

Good Machine Learning Practices (GMLP): Principles emphasizing the value of reproducibility, openness, and high-quality data [2].

7.2.4 International Perspectives

A risk-based framework for AI is proposed by the EU's Artificial Intelligence Act, with more stringent guidelines for high-risk applications such as medical diagnostics.

Draft rules for AI in healthcare, with an emphasis on data protection and responsibility, have also been released by China and Canada [3].

7.3 Patient Privacy and Data Security in AI Systems

7.3.1 Importance of Data in AI

Patient data, especially high-resolution photos and electronic medical records, is crucial to AI in dermatology. Such data presents serious privacy and security issues even if it is necessary for building reliable models [3].

7.3.2 Legal Frameworks

HIPAA (USA): Establishes guidelines for safeguarding private patient data.

Strict guidelines for data processing, access, and consent are established under the GDPR (EU) [3].

7.3.3 Risks and Vulnerabilities

Data Breaches: Cyberattacks may target centralized data storage.

Re-identification: In certain cases, especially in tiny datasets, even anonymized data might be linked to specific people.

Third-Party Access: If data governance is not well established, working with IT companies may provide hazards [4].

7.3.4 Mitigation Strategies

Anonymization and de-identification are methods for removing personal information from datasets.

Federated Learning: A decentralized method that removes the need to transport raw data between locations in order to train AI models.

Immutable records and transparent data access logs are provided by blockchain technology [4].

7.3.5 Ethical Considerations

Consent should be a continuous, open process, and patients should be informed about how their data is utilized. The ongoing application and advancement of AI in dermatology depend on trust [4].

7.4 Practical Considerations: Integrating AI into Clinical Practice

7.4.1 Clinician Training and Trust

Education: Dermatologists need to be aware of the constraints, outputs, and appropriate applications of AI.

Interpretability: To support clinical judgment, AI systems ought to offer justifications or confidence levels.

Building Trust: Gaining the trust of clinicians requires openness and proven accuracy [4].

7.4.2 Workflow Integration

User-Centered Design: AI systems ought to be easily incorporated into clinical procedures and current electronic health records (EHRs).

Decision Support: AI should support clinical judgment rather than take its place.

Clinical Feedback Loops: To enhance and customize AI recommendations, systems should accept feedback from clinicians [4].

7.4.3 Legal and Liability Issues

Responsibility: There is still some ambiguity over who is responsible for misdiagnosis involving AI.

Documentation: Accurate documentation of AI decision-making participation can aid in conflict resolution.

When using AI tools in patient care, patients should be informed in order to obtain their informed consent [5].

7.5 Economic and Infrastructural Barriers

Cost: For smaller clinics, high development and implementation expenses could be unaffordable.

Infrastructure: The operation of AI tools depends on dependable hardware, Internet, and IT support.

Payers are required to create reimbursement schemes that acknowledge the importance of diagnostics aided by AI [5].

7.5.1 Real-World Implementation

Successful integration case studies illustrate the possible advantages and difficulties of practical use, such as AI-based triage systems in teledermatology platforms or decision support in sizable dermatology clinics [5].

7.5.2 Summary

Dermatology could benefit much from AI, but its application needs to be carefully considered. To guarantee that emerging technologies enhance treatment for all patients without creating new dangers or inequities, ethical justice, robust legal frameworks, and workable integration mechanisms are crucial. The fundamental issues and proactive approaches required to appropriately adopt AI in the future of dermatological care have been outlined in this section.

References

1. Esteva A, Kuprel B, Novoa R, et al. Dermatologist-level classification of skin cancer with deep neural networks. Nature. 2017;542:115–8. https://doi.org/10.1038/nature21056.
2. Choi JY, Dawe R, Ibbotson S, Fleming C, Doney A, Foerster J. Quantitative analysis of topical treatments in atopic dermatitis: unexpectedly low use of emollients and strong correlation of topical corticosteroid use both with depression and concurrent asthma. Br J Dermatol. 2020;182(4):1017–25. https://doi.org/10.1111/bjd.18265.
3. Liu F-H. The antecedents and effects of manufacturer service innovation: A relationship-learning perspective. In: 2016 Portland International Conference on Management of Engineering and Technology (PICMET), Honolulu, HI, USA; 2016. p. 2959–69. https://doi.org/10.1109/PICMET.2016.7806811.
4. Rajkomar A, Oren E, Chen K, et al. Scalable and accurate deep learning with electronic health records. NPJ Digit Med. 2018;1:18. https://doi.org/10.1038/s41746-018-0029-1.
5. Rocher L, Hendrickx JM, de Montjoye YA. Estimating the success of re-identifications in incomplete datasets using generative models. Nat Commun. 2019;10:3069. https://doi.org/10.1038/s41467-019-10933-3.

AI and Future Directions in Dermatology

8

Esraa M. AlEdani

8.1 Personalized Dermatology Through AI

The goal of personalized medicine is to adjust treatment regimens to each patient's particular genetic, environmental, and behavioral characteristics. Through the analysis of massive datasets that include clinical imaging, genomes, proteomics, and patient history, artificial intelligence (AI) holds the potential to completely transform the discipline of dermatology. AI systems can offer a more thorough understanding of each illness presentation by combining such diverse data, which will ultimately lead to more precise diagnoses and individualized treatment plans [1].

Historically, clinical experience and textbook knowledge have played a major role in dermatological diagnosis and therapy. However, by spotting connections and patterns that the human eye cannot see, AI models can go far beyond these limitations. Clinicians may prescribe an alternate treatment in advance if a machine learning algorithm trained on thousands of patient data finds, for example, that a certain genetic mutation correlates with resistance to a common acne medicine [1].

AI-driven personalization in clinical contexts might include forecasting negative reactions to frequently administered dermatological drugs or suggesting tailored treatments for long-term ailments like psoriasis based on a patient's biomarker profile. Another potential area is the use of wearable technology that can continuously monitor the skin. Real-time data may be fed into AI systems via devices with cameras and sensors, which would then evaluate the course of the disease and make real-time therapy recommendations. These flexible, adaptable treatment programs

E. M. AlEdani (✉)
University of Basrah, College of Medicine, Basra, Iraq

E. M. AlEdani, H. I. Maibach (eds.), *Applications of Artificial Intelligence in Common Dermatological Diseases*, Updates in Clinical Dermatology,
https://doi.org/10.1007/978-3-031-78139-1_8

may greatly enhance patient outcomes and lessen the need for face-to-face appointments [1].

AI may also make it easier to create customized skincare regimens based on a person's hormone cycles, environmental exposures, and skin flora. AI systems could modify regimens over time to maximize effectiveness and minimize negative effects by utilizing patient-reported results and longitudinal data. AI-powered personalized dermatology aims to empower patients to actively understand and manage their own skin health in addition to optimizing treatments [1].

8.2 AI and Robotics in Skin Surgery and Treatment

There is increasing interest in using AI for therapy, particularly in procedural and surgical dermatology, even if the majority of its uses in dermatology are now focused on diagnostic tasks. There are intriguing opportunities to improve the accuracy, security, and accessibility of dermatological therapies at the nexus of artificial intelligence and robotics [2].

AI-enhanced imaging can assist in more precisely defining tumor margins during skin cancer operations, especially Mohs micrographic surgery, than traditional techniques. Real-time guidance during excision can be provided by machine learning algorithms trained on annotated histopathology slides, assisting surgeons in preventing both undertreatment and needless loss of healthy tissue. In addition to improving therapeutic results, this maintains aesthetic appeal, which is particularly crucial for facial procedures [2].

When paired with artificial intelligence, robotic devices can improve surgical precision by doing delicate or extremely repetitious operations with little variation. For instance, by adjusting the energy intensity and duration based on skin type, thickness, and real-time feedback from optical sensors, robots could help with laser treatments for vascular lesions, pigmentation problems, or acne scars. These systems have the potential to decrease the duration of procedures, minimize the likelihood of problems, and standardize the quality of care provided by various healthcare providers [3].

AI-powered robotics may be applied to chronic wound care in addition to surgery. In addition to applying dressings, delivering drugs, and warning physicians of infection or delayed healing, autonomous systems might evaluate the stages of wound healing. Such methods could greatly increase access to expert-level care in long-term care facilities or isolated areas with a shortage of dermatologists [3].

Additionally, AI-enabled robotic systems may improve cosmetic dermatology operations. Botulinum toxin injections, automated microneedling, and fillers with precise guidance from real-time skin imaging and mapping are a few examples of applications. These technologies have the potential to decrease human error, provide consistent outcomes for a range of patient demographics, and democratize access to high-quality dermatological procedures [3].

8.3 The Road Ahead: Opportunities and Limitations

Although there is a lot of promise for AI in dermatology, achieving its full potential will rely on how new issues are resolved. Increasing the accessibility of dermatological care via teledermatology platforms and AI-powered mobile applications is one of the biggest prospects. These technologies can provide diagnostic services to underserved or distant communities with a shortage of dermatologists. The strain on urban healthcare facilities could be lessened if patients had access to a smartphone and the internet for initial assessments and management guidance [4].

The creation of consumer-focused AI solutions for early skin cancer detection is another exciting avenue. Apps that can identify problematic lesions or moles for additional testing may promote earlier clinical visits and enhance the prognosis for diseases like melanoma. The incorporation of these more advanced instruments into daily skincare regimens may normalize preventative dermatology and promote consistent self-monitoring [4].

Nonetheless, a number of restrictions still exist. The problem of generalizability is the most important of these. AI models may not function well in a variety of contexts if they were trained on data from particular geographic areas, ethnic groups, or healthcare systems. This emphasizes how crucial it is to develop varied, inclusive, and uniform databases. Acceptance by clinicians is another issue. Dermatologists could be hesitant to use instruments that they don't understand or that they believe will undermine their knowledge. Strong clinical validation, transparent algorithms, and unambiguous performance measures are necessary to establish trust [4].

There are still unsolved ethical and legal issues as well. With mistakes in dermatology having the potential to have both psychological and medical repercussions, concerns over the proper degree of autonomy to be given to AI systems are especially urgent. What about legal accountability in the case of a misdiagnosis caused by AI? Updated legislative frameworks and cooperative stakeholder interactions are required to answer these issues [5].

Economically speaking, major expenditures in infrastructure, maintenance, and training will be required for the integration of AI and robotics into dermatology. Without government funding or public-private partnerships, adoption may be difficult for smaller clinics and practices. Since AI-assisted consultations and procedures have the potential to lower long-term healthcare costs by increasing diagnostic precision and treatment effectiveness, reimbursement models will need to change to take this into account [5].

To increase the interpretability, flexibility, and security of AI systems, ongoing technological improvements are needed. Present-day deep learning models frequently operate as "black boxes," making it challenging for medical professionals to comprehend the logic underlying certain results. Explainable AI (XAI) should be given top priority in future advancements in order to boost clinician confidence and make incorporation into clinical decision-making easier [5].

Collaboration across disciplines will be essential to all of these initiatives. For AI systems to be clinically useful, morally sound, and socially responsible, developers must collaborate closely with dermatologists, ethicists, patients, and legislators. Furthermore, the establishment of worldwide standards for the development and application of AI in dermatology would require international cooperation [5].

8.4 Conclusion

AI's use in dermatology is expected to grow significantly beyond its current uses as it develops further. AI has the potential to revolutionize everything from robotic-assisted procedures that improve accuracy and efficiency to individualized treatment programs based on genetic and environmental data. However, continued efforts in validation, regulation, and interdisciplinary cooperation are necessary for this future to be responsibly achieved. AI in dermatology holds great promise for improving care, equality, and outcomes for all patients through innovation based on ethics and data. This promise is not just technological but also deeply human.

References

1. Kololgi SP, Lahari CS. Harnessing the power of artificial intelligence in dermatology: a comprehensive commentary. Indian J Dermatol. 2023;68(6):678–81. https://doi.org/10.4103/ijd.ijd_581_23. Epub 2024 Jan 9. PMID: 38371574; PMCID: PMC10868991.
2. Li Z, Koban KC, Schenck TL, Giunta RE, Li Q, Sun Y. Artificial intelligence in dermatology image analysis: current developments and future trends. J Clin Med. 2022;11(22):6826. https://doi.org/10.3390/jcm11226826. PMID: 36431301; PMCID: PMC9693628.
3. Kassir M, Goldust M. Robotic-assisted procedures in cosmetic dermatology. J Cosmet Dermatol. 2024;23(11):3774–5. https://doi.org/10.1111/jocd.16551. Epub 2024 Sep 12. PMID: 39267251.
4. Omiye JA, Gui H, Daneshjou R, Cai ZR, Muralidharan V. Principles, applications, and future of artificial intelligence in dermatology. Front Med (Lausanne). 2023;10:1278232. https://doi.org/10.3389/fmed.2023.1278232. PMID: 37901399; PMCID: PMC10602645.
5. Liopyris K, Gregoriou S, Dias J, Stratigos AJ. Artificial intelligence in dermatology: challenges and perspectives. Dermatol Ther (Heidelb). 2022;12(12):2637–51. https://doi.org/10.1007/s13555-022-00833-8. Epub 2022 Oct 28. PMID: 36306100; PMCID: PMC9674813.

Index

E. M. AlEdani, H. I. Maibach (eds.), *Applications of Artificial Intelligence in Common Dermatological Diseases*, Updates in Clinical Dermatology, https://doi.org/10.1007/978-3-031-78139-1

GPSR Compliance

The European Union's (EU) General Product Safety Regulation (GPSR) is a set of rules that requires consumer products to be safe and our obligations to ensure this.

If you have any concerns about our products, you can contact us on ProductSafety@springernature.com

In case Publisher is established outside the EU, the EU authorized representative is:

Springer Nature Customer Service Center GmbH
Europaplatz 3
69115 Heidelberg, Germany

Batch number: 10732107

Printed by Printforce, the Netherlands